Lecture Notes
in Business Information Processing   359

Series Editors

Wil van der Aalst
  RWTH Aachen University, Aachen, Germany
John Mylopoulos
  University of Trento, Trento, Italy
Michael Rosemann
  Queensland University of Technology, Brisbane, QLD, Australia
Michael J. Shaw
  University of Illinois, Urbana-Champaign, IL, USA
Clemens Szyperski
  Microsoft Research, Redmond, WA, USA

More information about this series at http://www.springer.com/series/7911

Stanisław Wrycza · Jacek Maślankowski (Eds.)

Information Systems: Research, Development, Applications, Education

12th SIGSAND/PLAIS EuroSymposium 2019
Gdansk, Poland, September 19, 2019
Proceedings

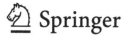 Springer

Editors
Stanisław Wrycza🆔
Department of Business Informatics
University of Gdansk
Gdansk, Poland

Jacek Maślankowski🆔
Department of Business Informatics
University of Gdansk
Gdansk, Poland

ISSN 1865-1348   ISSN 1865-1356 (electronic)
Lecture Notes in Business Information Processing
ISBN 978-3-030-29607-0   ISBN 978-3-030-29608-7 (eBook)
https://doi.org/10.1007/978-3-030-29608-7

This Springer imprint is published by the registered company Springer Nature Switzerland AG
The registered company address is: Gewerbestrasse 11, 6330 Cham, Switzerland

Preface

EuroSymposium is already in its 12th edition. This cyclical, annual event has been changing and extending its thematic scope in accordance with the rapid progress being made within the field of Information Systems knowledge and applications, with its currently emerging areas, in the era of the digital transformation. The new topics fall within the sphere of social networks analytics, mobile systems, Internet of Things, Big Data, Machine Learning, Industry 4.0, User Experience, and several others. All of them have the strong influence on the EuroSymposium subject matter, changing it fundamentally as compared with the first EuroSymposia.

The objective of the SIGSAND/PLAIS EuroSymposium 2019 is to promote and develop high-quality research on all issues related to research, development, applications, and education of Information Systems (IS), often referred to in Europe as Business Informatics. It provided a forum for IS researchers and practitioners in Europe and beyond to interact, collaborate, and develop this field. The EuroSymposia were initiated by Prof. Keng Siau as the SIGSAND – Europe Initiative. Previous EuroSymposia were held at:

- University of Galway, Ireland, 2006
- University of Gdansk, Poland, 2007
- University of Marburg, Germany, 2008
- University of Gdansk, Poland, 2011–2018

The accepted papers of the EuroSymposia held in Gdansk have been published in:

- 2nd EuroSymposium 2007: Bajaj, A., Wrycza, S. (eds.): Systems analysis and design for advanced modeling methods: best practices, information science reference, IGI Global, Hershey, New York (2009)
- 4th EuroSymposium 2011: Wrycza, S. (ed.): Research in Systems Analysis and Design: Models and Methods. LNBIP, vol. 93, Springer, Berlin (2011)
- Joint Working Conferences EMMSAD/EuroSymposium 2012 held at CAiSE 2012: Bider, I., Halpin, T., Krogstie, J., Nurcan, S., Proper, E., Schmidt, R., Soffer, P., Wrycza, S. (eds.): Enterprise, Business-Process and Information Systems Modeling. LNBIP, vol. 113, Springer, Berlin (2012)
- 6th SIGSAND/PLAIS EuroSymposium 2013: Wrycza, S. (ed.): Information Systems: Development, Learning, Security. LNBIP, vol. 161, Springer, Berlin (2013)
- 7th SIGSAND/PLAIS EuroSymposium 2014: Wrycza, S. (ed.): Information Systems: Education, Applications, Research. LNBIP, vol. 193, Springer, Berlin (2014)
- 8th SIGSAND/PLAIS EuroSymposium 2015: Wrycza, S. (ed.): Information Systems: Development, Applications, Education. LNBIP, vol. 232, Springer, Berlin (2015)
- 9th SIGSAND/PLAIS EuroSymposium 2016: Wrycza, S. (ed.): Information Systems: Development, Research, Applications, Education. LNBIP, vol. 264, Springer, Berlin (2016)

- 10th Jubilee SIGSAND/PLAIS EuroSymposium 2017: Wrycza, S., Maślankowski, J. (eds.): Information Systems: Development, Research, Applications, Education. LNBIP, vol. 300, Springer, Berlin (2017)
- 11th SIGSAND/PLAIS EuroSymposium 2018: Wrycza, S., Maślankowski, J. (eds.): Information Systems: Research, Development, Applications, Education. LNBIP, vol. 333, Springer, Berlin (2018)

There were three organizers of the 12th EuroSymposium on Systems Analysis and Design:

- PLAIS – Polish Chapter of AIS
- SIGSAND – Special Interest Group on Systems Analysis and Design of AIS
- Department of Business Informatics of University of Gdansk, Poland

The Polish Chapter of Association for Information Systems (PLAIS) was established in 2006 as the joint initiative of Prof. Claudia Loebbecke, former President of AIS, and Prof. Stanislaw Wrycza, University of Gdansk, Poland. PLAIS co-organizes international and domestic IS conferences and has gained the title of Outstanding Chapter of the Association for Information Systems for years 2014, 2016, 2017, and 2018.

SIGSAND is one of the most active SIGs with quite substantial record of contributions for AIS. It provides services such as annual American and European Symposia on SIGSAND, research and teaching tracks at major IS conferences, listserv, and special issues in journals.

The Department of Business Informatics of University of Gdansk conducts the intensive teaching and research activities. Some of its academic books are bestsellers in Poland (recently, "Business Informatics. Theory and Applications," PWN Publisher, 2019, 863 pages, in Polish) and the department is also active internationally. Recently, the leading areas of the department's scholars research and publishing in international academic IS journals are: unified theory of acceptance and use of technology, as well as Information Technology occupational culture ITOC. The most significant conference organized by the department was: the Xth European Conference on Information Systems (ECIS 2002). The department is a partner of ERCIS consortium – European Research Center for Information Systems and SAP University Alliances SUA. The students of Business Informatics of University of Gdansk have been awarded several times for their innovative projects at the annual AIS Student Chapters Competition in the USA.

EuroSymposium 2019 received 32 papers from 13 different countries. The submission and review process was supported by the Open Conference System (OCS) hosted by Springer. The members of international Program Committee carefully evaluated the submissions, selecting 12 papers for publication in this LNBIP volume. Therefore, EuroSymposium 2019 had an acceptance rate of 37%, with submissions divided into the following four groups:

- Information Systems in Business
- Health Informatics and Life-Long-Learning
- IT Security
- Agile Methods and Software Engineering

The keynote speech entitled "Engaging Practitioners in IS Research Through Action Design Research," was given by Prof. Matti Rossi from Aalto University of Business, Finland.

I would like to express my thanks to all Authors, Reviewers, Advisory Board, International Programme Committee and Organizational Committee members for their support, efforts, and time. They have made possible the successful accomplishment of EuroSymposium 2019.

Stanisław Wrycza

Organization

General Chair

Stanislaw Wrycza   University of Gdansk, Poland

Organizers

- The Polish Chapter of Association for Information Systems - PLAIS
- SIGSAND is the Association for Information Systems (AIS) Special Interest Group on Systems Analysis and Design
- Department of Business Informatics at University of Gdansk

Advisory Board

Wil van der Aalst	RWTH Aachen University, Germany
David Avison	ESSEC Business School, France
Joerg Becker	European Research Centre for Information Systems, Germany
Jane Fedorowicz	Bentley University, USA
Alan Hevner	University of South Florida, USA
Claudia Loebbecke	University of Cologne, Germany
Keng Siau	Missouri University of Science and Technology, USA
Roman Słowinski	Chairman of the Committee on Informatics of the Polish Academy of Sciences, Poland

International Program Committee

Özlem Albayrak	Turkey
Eduard Babkin	National Research University, Russia
Witold Chmielarz	University of Warsaw, Poland
Helena Dudycz	Wroclaw University of Economics, Poland
Peter Forbrig	University of Rostock, Germany
Piotr Jedrzejowicz	Gdynia Maritime University, Poland
Bjoern Johansson	Lund University, Sweden
Kalinka Kaloyanova	Sofia University, Bulgaria
Jolanta Kowal	University of Wroclaw, Poland
Henryk Krawczyk	Gdansk University of Technology, Poland
Kyootai Lee	Sogang University, Korea
Tim A. Majchrzak	University of Agder, Norway
Ngoc-Thanh Nguyen	University of Wroclaw, Poland
Nikolaus Obwegeser	Aarhus University, Denmark

Mieczyslaw L. Owoc	Wroclaw University of Economics, Poland
Joanna Paliszkiewicz	Warsaw University of Life Sciences, Poland
Malgorzata Pankowska	Katowice University of Economics, Poland
Marian Niedzwiedziński	University of Computer Science and Skills, Poland
Nava Pliskin	Ben-Gurion University of the Negev, Israel
Isabel Ramos	The University of Minho, Portugal
Michael Rosemann	Queensland University of Technology, Australia
Thomas Schuster	Pforzheim University, Germany
Janice C. Sipior	Villanova University, USA
Andrzej Sobczak	Warsaw School of Economics, Poland
Piotr Soja	Cracow University of Economics, Poland
Jakub Swacha	University of Szczecin, Poland
Pere Tumbas	University of Novi Sad, Serbia
Catalin Vrabie	National University, Romania
Yinglin Wang	Shanghai University of Finance and Economics, China
H. Roland Weistroffer	Virginia Commonwealth University, USA
Carson Woo	Sauder School of Business, Canada
Iryna Zolotaryova	Kharkiv National University of Economics, Ukraine

Organizing Committee

Chair

Stanislaw Wrycza (President of Polish Chapter of AIS (PLAIS))	University of Gdansk, Poland

Secretary

Anna Węsierska	University of Gdansk, Poland

Members

Michał Kuciapski (Secretary of Polish Chapter of AIS (PLAIS))	University of Gdansk, Poland
Jacek Maślankowski	University of Gdansk, Poland
Dorota Buchnowska	University of Gdansk, Poland
Bartłomiej Gawin	University of Gdansk, Poland
Przemysław Jatkiewicz	University of Gdansk, Poland
Dariusz Kralewski	University of Gdansk, Poland
Bartosz Marcinkowski	University of Gdansk, Poland

Patronage

- European Research Center for Information Systems (ERCIS)
- Committee on Informatics of the Polish Academy of Sciences

EuroSymposium 2019 Topics

Agile Methods
Big Data, Business Analytics
Blockchain Technology and Applications
Business Informatics
Business Process Modeling
Case Studies in SAND
Cloud Computing
Cognitive Issues in SAND
Conceptual Modeling
Crowdsourcing and Crowdfunding Models
Design Science
Digital Services and Social Media
Enterprise Architecture
Enterprise Social Networks
ERP and CRM Systems
Ethical and Human Aspects of IS Development
Ethnographic, Anthropological, Action and Entrepreneurial Research
Evolution of IS Discipline
Human-Computer Interaction
Industry 4.0
Information Systems Development: Methodologies, Methods, Techniques and Tools
Internet of Things
Machine Learning
Model-Driven Architecture
New Paradigms, Formalisms, Approaches, Frameworks and Challenges in IS & SAND
Ontological Foundations and Intelligent Systems of SAND
Open Source Software (OSS) Solutions
Project Management
Quality Assurance in Systems Development, DevOps
Requirements and Software Engineering
Research Methodologies in SAND
Role of SAND in Mobile and Internet Applications Development
SAND Education: Curricula, E-learning, MOOCs and Teaching Cases
SCRUM Approach
Security and Privacy Issues in IS & SAND
Service Oriented Systems Development
Social Networking Services

Socio-Technical Approaches to System Development, Psychological and Behavioural
   Descriptions
Software Intensive Systems and Services
Strategic Information Systems in Enterprises
Supply Chain Management Aspects
Systems Analysts and Designers Professions
Teams and Teamwork in IS & SAND
UML, SysML, BPMN
User Experience (UX) Design
Workflow Management

Contents

Information Systems in Business

Introducing Knowledge Graphs to Decision Support Systems Design. 3
  Samaa Elnagar and Heinz Roland Weistroffer

Reducing Consultant Information Asymmetry in Enterprise System
Implementation Projects - The Transaction Cost Economics View. 12
  Przemysław Lech

A Study of the Impact of Internal and External Usability on Knowledge
Transfer by the Means of Mobile Technologies: Preliminary Results 20
  Paweł Weichbroth and Michał Kuciapski

Health Informatics and Life-Long-Learning

Model-Based Diagnosis with FTTell: Assessing the Potential for Pediatric
Failure to Thrive (FTT) During the Perinatal Stage 37
  Natali Levi-Soskin, Ron Shaoul, Hanan Kohen, Ahmad Jbara,
  and Dov Dori

Supporting Active and Healthy Ageing by ICT Solutions: Preliminary
Lessons Learned from Polish, Swedish and Latvian Older Adults 48
  Ewa Soja, Piotr Soja, Ella Kolkowska, and Marite Kirikova

3D Authoring Tool for Blended Learning. 62
  Andrew Zaliwski and Karishma Kelsey

IT Security

DevSecOps Metrics. 77
  Luís Prates, João Faustino, Miguel Silva, and Rúben Pereira

Enculturation of Cyber Safety Awareness for Communities in South Africa . . . 91
  Dorothy Scholtz and Elmarie Kritzinger

Privacy Concerns and Remedies in Mobile Recommender Systems (MRSs). . . 105
  Ramandeep Kaur Sandhu, Heinz Roland Weistroffer,
  and Josephine Stanley-Brown

Agile Methods and Software Engineering

Towards Agile Architecting: Proposing an Architectural Pathway Within
an Industry 4.0 Project.   121
  Nuno Santos, Nuno Ferreira, and Ricardo J. Machado

Towards Model-Driven Role Engineering in BPM Software Systems.   137
  Eduard Babkin, Pavel Malyzhenkov, and Constantine Yavorskiy

Communication and Documentation Practices in Agile Requirements
Engineering: A Survey in Polish Software Industry   147
  Aleksander Jarzębowicz and Natalia Sitko

Author Index   159

Information Systems in Business

Introducing Knowledge Graphs to Decision Support Systems Design

Samaa Elnagar[(⊠)] and Heinz Roland Weistroffer[(⊠)]

Virigina Commonwealth University, Richmond, VA, USA
{elnagarsa, hrweistr}@vcu.edu

Abstract. Recent progress in cognitive technologies has driven *decision support system (DSS)* development in more complex directions. One of the main challenges in efficient DSS design is knowledge acquisition, especially in complicated and uncertain decision contexts. The more knowledge available to the system, the better decisions can be generated by a DSS. Representation of knowledge plays an important role in finding solutions to problems. With advances in the *Semantic Web*, knowledge can be represented in structured formats such as ontologies, which ease search and reasoning tasks. However, new data cannot be easily integrated nor updated in ontologies in real-time. Consequently, *knowledge graphs (KGs)* have emerged as a dynamic, scalable and domain independent form of knowledge representation. This paper explores how KGs can enhance the decision-making process in DSSs. Moreover, the paper presents a framework that may facilitate the integration of KGs into the DSS design.

Keywords: Decision support systems · Knowledge graphs ·
Knowledge integration · Ontologies · Timeliness

1 Introduction

A DSS as an intelligent system should be able to evolve through adaptive development [1]. Intelligent systems evolution depends primarily on new knowledge acquisition. Knowledge can have a profound effect on professional decision-making [2]. While a firm comprises individuals and a set of definable objectified resources, its most strategically important feature is its body of collective knowledge. A firm's first advantage in today's business environment is its ability to leverage and utilize its knowledge [3]. Knowledge stored in intelligent DSSs comes from heterogeneous data sources such as databases, knowledge bases, and external sources of mostly unstructured data. However, many organizations suffer from underutilization of the available knowledge because it is hard to process and integrate heterogeneous unstructured data [4]. In addition to the lack or underutilization of knowledge, efficient decision support is complicated by multifaceted and indeterminate decision situations.

In order for DSSs to evolve, real-time updates of knowledge are needed, taking into consideration the organizational decision-making position. The difficulty of keeping the knowledge up-to-date in the organizational memory is one of the main hindrances to the automatic evolution of DSS [5]. Thus, knowledge timeliness is an important

© Springer Nature Switzerland AG 2019
S. Wrycza and J. Maślankowski (Eds.): SIGSAND/PLAIS 2019, LNBIP 359, pp. 3–11, 2019.
https://doi.org/10.1007/978-3-030-29608-7_1

challenge in efficient decision support. Another significant challenge to be addressed is the appropriate representation of knowledge that facilitates search, retrieval and inference processes. Semantic Web technologies aim to represent knowledge in structured formats in the form of concepts and relations [6].

Ontologies have emerged as a semantic representation of domain knowledge. Ontologies have been used extensively in DSS to ease the retrieval and interpretation of knowledge. The strength of ontologies lies in their semantic power that facilitates the reasoning and inference of knowledge [7]. However, ontologies are domain dependent and require domain engineers to build and maintain, in addition to cost and time [8]. Moreover, new knowledge is hard to integrate with existing domain ontologies, especially if they encompass cross domain knowledge [9, 10]. Timeliness is also an issue in ontologies. Since most updates in ontologies are done manually by domain experts [11], there will be times that an ontology is incomplete.

Knowledge graphs (KGs) have emerged as possible answers to the limitations of ontologies. KGs generators turn unstructured data into a structured knowledge format for a domain-specific or domain independent situation [12]. In comparison to other semantic representations of knowledge, knowledge graphs have salient features of real-time knowledge representation structures, information management processes, and search and reasoning algorithms [13]. The scalability, timeliness and data integrity of KGs makes them the backbone for many intelligent systems and many enterprise systems [14].

Using KGs in DSSs allows links between information and content sources that might not otherwise be easily identified as related. KGs enhance the efficacy of content management through allowing real-time updates of knowledge and easy search and retrieval tasks. KGs can be used by machine learning systems to document their decision flows and add more transparency to the *Artificial Intelligence (AI)* decision-making process [15]. This paper investigates how KGs can enhance the efficiency and the performance of DSSs. In addition, the paper proposes a simple framework that shows how KGs can be embedded in existing DSSs without significantly changing the DSS design. This framework may help organizations enhance the efficiency of existing DSSs with minimal effort and cost.

2   Knowledge Graphs Advantages and Limitations

KGs were developed as extensions for linked open data and were first introduced by Google in 2012 (Google Knowledge Graph). Ehrlinger and Wöß [16] define knowledge graphs as "large networks of entities, their semantic types, properties, and relationships between entities". KGs are generated at runtime using automatic KG generators such as *IBM Watson, Siri, and Neo4j* [17]. Thus, data timeliness is insured in KGs [11]. One of the greatest values of KGs is that they are inherently explainable because they explicitly identify all entities and their relationships [15]. For example: KGs can uncover facts that would be extremely arduous to find using traditional methods. Figure 1[1] represents the

---

[1] The figure was generated using NEO4j sandbox.

KG of some of the crimes occurred in Manchester UK in August 2017. Officer Ber and Shamus (the blue nodes) reported the same type of crime in two different places in two days in a row. Investigating the relations between the two crimes using the knowledge graph we can see that Kathleen, who was investigated by officer Shamus, knows Alan, who performed the second crime. In addition, Kathleen and Alan (the orange nodes) know Jack who performed the same type of crime. Further investigation revealed that the three criminals were affiliated to the same crime group. Without the KG, it would have been harder to discover the relation between the two crimes or to discover the relations to the third crime.

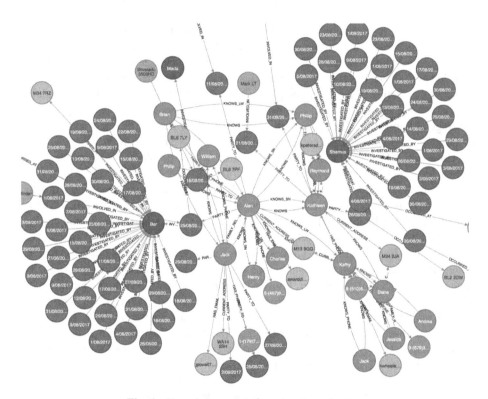

Fig. 1. Knowledge graph for crime investigation

To capture the equivalent knowledge using ontologies, four main ontologies would be needed as shown in Fig. 2. Ontologies focus more on the structure and properties of each class in a hierarchal form, which makes integrating the knowledge in each ontology a tedious process. Moreover, displaying the relations between instances in an ontology does not require processing of knowledge in the same form as in a KG.

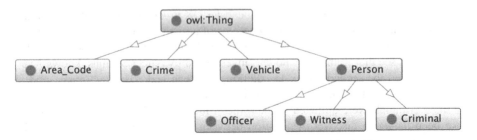

Fig. 2. Ontology with equivalent basic classes as in the KG of Fig. 1.

KGs are very useful in data integration tasks because they can be scaled to different data sizes and levels of heterogeneity. While ontologies define all concepts and relations for a certain domain, KG schemas contain the entities and relations of the knowledge in hand. In contrast to ontologies, KGs are generated based on the entities found in the corpus. Therefore, completeness is a main challenge to KGs. Completeness issues are associated with an entity having all expected attributes [18]. So, the coverage of knowledge graphs, as well as their efficiency must be ensured while in use. In addition, reasoning and inference capabilities of KGs are very high.

However, KGs are not the perfect solution to all problems. The quality of a knowledge graph is crucial for its applications, but the quality of KGs is always questionable [19]. The quality of the generated KGs is highly dependent on the quality of the data sources [20]. For example, the quality of a KG generated from an encyclopedia is generally higher than the quality of a KG generated from social media. Consequently, it is likely that KGs may be incorrect [21]. Moreover, the larger a KG, the harder it is to maintain it. Usually KGs are maintained using human intervention to ensure their quality [22]. KGs should be consistent and not contain conflicting or contradictory data [23]. Moreover, knowledge graphs are hard to compare against each other in a given setting [24]. Security and privacy is also a concern in KGs [25]. A summary of the advantages and limitations of KGs are shown in Table 1.

To overcome the limitations of KGs, generated KGs must be refined in terms of *incompleteness, incorrectness (fault tolerance), coverage, and inconsistency*. For further information, please refer to [22] and [12].

Table 1. Knowledge graph advantages and limitations

Advantages	Limitations
Scalability	Incomplete
Problem specific	Shallow domain knowledge
Timeliness	Inconsistent with domain knowledge
Automatic generation	Usually incorrect
Easy data integration	Not trustworthy
Agile	*Redundant*
Easy evolution	*Hard to compare*
Machine and human friendly	*Challenging maintenance*
Evolution	*Low interoperability*
Reasoning power	*Security is questionable*

3 Related Work

Liu et al. [26] developed a methodology to evaluate stock news sentiment market by using the enterprise knowledge graph embedding that systematically considers various types of relationships between listed stocks. The system uses the *Gated Recurrent Unit (GRU)* model to combine the correlated stocks' news sentiment and the focal stock's quantitative features to predict the focal stock's price movement.

Singh et al. [15] developed *KNADIA*, a conversational dialogue system for intra-enterprise use, providing knowledge-assisted question answering and transactional assistance to employees of a large organization. The system uses conversational agents (bots) to answer users' queries based on information stored in KG. Another approach is followed in the *RdfLiveNews* prototype, where RSS web feeds of news companies are used to address the aspect of timeliness in *DBpedia*, i.e., extracting new information that is either outdated or missing in *DBpedia* [27].

KGs could also empower sales and marketing teams to locate content that is related to whatever their current needs are, and locate the content tagged files appropriately [28]. Shi et al. [29] proposed a model to integrate heterogeneous textual medical knowledge with health data, which can support semantic querying and reasoning. They developed a knowledge retrieval framework to transform the textual knowledge into machine-readable format, by constructing a semantic health KG.

4 How to Use KGs in Decision Support

Knowledge sources are fundamental elements in designing DSSs. For efficient exchange of knowledge amongst the decision makers, the facilitation of structured language and the representation of knowledge are important objectives. *Enterprise Knowledge Graphs (EKGs)* have emerged as a collection of tools and a back-end infrastructure used by enterprises for creating custom, domain-specific Knowledge Graphs [30]. In other words, an EKG is an industry-specific KG that represents all the concepts and relations needed for a certain enterprise or industry. Knowledge sources could be of good quality such as knowledge bases and databases or of questionable quality such as online web data sources. EKGs can be constructed by integrating a few separate KGs from different data sources with schema alignment and instancing matching mechanisms.

Since enterprise terminologies are aligned with standardized metadata, enterprise data may be interlinked and easily reused by other departments [25]. The expected quality of the EKG should be evaluated before it is used in a DSS. The benefits of EKGs to DSSs can be summarized as follows:

- EKGs can help the decision-making process in ill-structured problems. Regarding the efficiency of DSSs, EKGs may speed up the response time and enhance the confidence in the answers.
- EKGs can facilitate the reasoning and inference tasks of DSSs. EKGs are stored in *RDF (resource description framework)* format and semantic search and retrieval processes are performed using the *SPARQL* language [11].
- EKGs allow real-time analytics because EKGs ensure zero latency and real-time performance, regardless of the number or depth of relationships.

In the next section we discuss in details the proposed framework that shows how EKGs can be embedded in DSSs.

5   The Proposed Framework Design

This framework aims to integrate EKGs into DSSs without changing the main foundational modules of DSSs. The main components of a DSS are knowledge sources, data models, inference engines, and the user interface [31]. In this framework, a new module is added for EKG generation and utilization as shown in Fig. 3.

5.1   Knowledge Module

This module contains all the knowledge sources that may be useful in the decision-making process. The knowledge can exist in structured formats such as databases and knowledge bases or in unstructured formats such as free texts in documents, online data sources and *RSS (Rich Site Summary)* feeds.

5.2   Knowledge Graph Generation Module

In this module the knowledge from different data source are fed into the KG generator to generate a knowledge graph that represents the enterprise related knowledge, i.e. a domain specific knowledge graph or enterprise knowledge graph (EKG).

5.2.1   KG Generator

Usually KG generators use complicated machine-learning methods, natural language processing, and inference techniques to create concepts and relations from the selected corpus in the form of RDF triples. As KG generators are very complex and time and

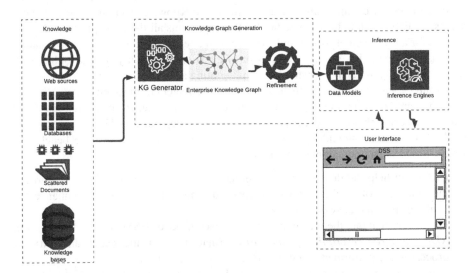

Fig. 3. Framework for integrating knowledge graphs in decision support systems

labor extensive, some companies use third-party services to generate KGs such as *Neo4j and IBM Watson*. KGs are generated automatically at runtime, to ensure timeliness of data and instant updates of knowledge.

5.2.2 In-House or Third Party

On the one hand, building knowledge graphs from scratch is a tedious and very complex proposition. On the other hand, third-party systems already offer good quality KGs generation services at reasonable cost. However, using third party systems may raise privacy and reliability concerns [25]. Thus, organizations need to make a tradeoff between building their own KGs or using emerging industry-specific KGs produced by third parties. In other words, the time and effort spent to produce a KG should be weighed against the value and cost reduction of third party generators.

5.2.3 EKG

The generated KG is considered the organization's own ontology or EKG because it represents all the active knowledge that exist in the organizational memory, including external sources. The generated EKG has two representations. The first is a schema representation or *(T-Box)* that contains the classes and relations between classes. The second is an instance representation or *(A-Box)* that contains instances of the schema classes and relationships between instances.

Because the knowledge source used in generating KGs contains untrusted online sources, refinement of any KG is necessary to avoid data quality limitations in KGs. For KG completion, semantic matching models and translational distance models [32] are used to complete missing concepts and relations from the generated EKG using reference knowledge graphs such as DBPedia and Freebase [26]. Other refinement tasks include correcting false concepts and relations from the EKG.

5.3 Inference Module

In this module, two components are responsible for the reasoning tasks in the DSS:

Data Models: These are responsible for encoding knowledge, and producing frames, production rules, and semantic networks.

Inference Engines: In this component, reasoning approaches are used to select the best decision based on available knowledge. Reasoning approaches in DSSs include: similarity matching, probabilistic reasoning, logic-based reasoning, and reasoning based on machine learning [33]. While the most challenging reasoning approach is machine learning, KGs can solve the black box problem by tracing decision flows. *SPARQL* is used as the main querying language to search and retrieve facts from EKGs.

5.4 User Interface

In this component, interactions between users and the DSS are conducted. The user input to the system is "the problem" which is interpreted and formulated into a set of questions and queries.

6 Conclusion

Decision support systems are getting more complex. DSSs should automatically evolve to incorporate changes in available knowledge and the environment in order to better be able to solve complex and multifaceted problems. Knowledge Graphs embody a new methodology in representing data in a structured format. KGs are generated at runtime so they meet timeliness and data integration of new knowledge requirements. This paper explores the potential application of KGs in DSSs and also suggests a framework to guide organizations toward integrating KGs in the design of DSSs, without changing the main structure of the DSS design. Future work will include implementing and evaluating the framework in terms of data quality and performance.

References

1. Keen, P.G.: Decision support systems: a research perspective. In: Decision Support Systems: Issues and Challenges: Proceedings of an International Task Force Meeting (1980)
2. Tester, J.W., et al.: The future of geothermal energy. In: Impact of Enhanced Geothermal Systems (EGS) on the United States in the 21st Century, Massachusetts Institute of Technology, Cambridge, vol. 372 (2006)
3. Spender, J.C., Grant, R.M.: Knowledge and the firm: overview. Strateg. Manag. J. **17**(S2), 5–9 (1996)
4. Damodaran, L., Olphert, W.: Barriers and facilitators to the use of knowledge management systems. Behav. Inf. Technol. **19**(6), 405–413 (2000)
5. Sagalowicz, D.: Using personal data bases for decision support. In: IIASA Proceedings Series (1976)
6. Presutti, V., d'Amato, C., Gandon, F., d'Aquin, M., Staab, S., Tordai, A. (eds.): ESWC 2014. LNCS, vol. 8465. Springer, Cham (2014). https://doi.org/10.1007/978-3-319-07443-6
7. Lan, M., Xu, J., Gao, W.: Ontology feature extraction via vector learning algorithm and applied to similarity measuring and ontology mapping. IAENG Int. J. Comput. Sci. **43**(1), 10–19 (2016)
8. Gruber, T.R.: Toward principles for the design of ontologies used for knowledge sharing? Int. J. Hum. Comput. Stud. **43**(5–6), 907–928 (1995)
9. Schulz, S., et al.: Strengths and limitations of formal ontologies in the biomedical domain. Revista electronica de comunicacao, informacao inovacao em saude: RECIIS **3**(1), 31 (2009)
10. Pfaff, M., Neubig, S., Krcmar, H.: Ontology for semantic data integration in the domain of IT benchmarking. J. Data Seman. **7**(1), 29–46 (2018)
11. Galkin, M., Auer, S., Scerri, S.: Enterprise knowledge graphs: a backbone of linked enterprise data. In: 2016 IEEE/WIC/ACM International Conference on Web Intelligence (WI). IEEE (2016)
12. Paulheim, H.: Knowledge graph refinement: a survey of approaches and evaluation methods. Seman. Web **8**(3), 489–508 (2017)
13. Gomez-Perez, J.M., Pan, J.Z., Vetere, G., Wu, H.: Enterprise knowledge graph: an introduction. In: Pan, J., Vetere, G., Gomez-Perez, J., Wu, H. (eds.) Exploiting Linked Data and Knowledge Graphs in Large Organisations, pp. 1–14. Springer, Cham (2017). https://doi.org/10.1007/978-3-319-45654-6_1
14. Zaveri, A., et al.: Quality assessment for linked data: a survey. Seman. Web **7**(1), 63–93 (2016)
15. Singh, M., et al.: KNADIA: enterprise KNowledge Assisted DIAlogue systems using deep learning. In: 2018 IEEE 34th International Conference on Data Engineering (ICDE). IEEE (2018)

16. Ehrlinger, L., Wöß, W.: Towards a definition of knowledge graphs. In: SEMANTiCS (Posters, Demos, SuCCESS), vol. 48 (2016)
17. Hong, S., Park, N., Chakraborty, T., Kang, H., Kwon, S.: PAGE: answering graph pattern queries via knowledge graph embedding. In: Chin, F.Y.L., Chen, C.L.P., Khan, L., Lee, K., Zhang, L.-J. (eds.) BIGDATA 2018. LNCS, vol. 10968, pp. 87–99. Springer, Cham (2018). https://doi.org/10.1007/978-3-319-94301-5_7
18. Nishioka, C., Scherp, A.: Information-theoretic analysis of entity dynamics on the linked open data cloud. In: CEUR Workshop Proceedings. CEUR Workshop Proceedings (2016)
19. Pernelle, N., et al.: RDF data evolution: efficient detection and semantic representation of changes. In: Semantic Systems-SEMANTiCS2016, 4 p. (2016)
20. Bordes, A., Gabrilovich, E.: Constructing and mining web-scale knowledge graphs: KDD 2014 tutorial. In: Proceedings of the 20th ACM SIGKDD International Conference on Knowledge Discovery and Data Mining. ACM (2014)
21. Paulheim, H., Bizer, C.: Improving the quality of linked data using statistical distributions. Int. J. Seman. Web Inf. Syst. (IJSWIS) **10**(2), 63–86 (2014)
22. Rashid, M.R.A., et al.: Completeness and consistency analysis for evolving knowledge bases. J. Web Seman. **54**, 48–71 (2019)
23. Paulheim, H., Stuckenschmidt, H.: Fast approximate a-box consistency checking using machine learning. In: Sack, H., Blomqvist, E., d'Aquin, M., Ghidini, C., Ponzetto, S.P., Lange, C. (eds.) ESWC 2016. LNCS, vol. 9678, pp. 135–150. Springer, Cham (2016). https://doi.org/10.1007/978-3-319-34129-3_9
24. Färber, M., et al.: Linked data quality of DBpedia, Freebase, OpenCyc, Wikidata, and YAGO. Seman. Web **9**(1), 77–129 (2018)
25. Ruan, T., Xue, L., Wang, H., Hu, F., Zhao, L., Ding, J.: Building and exploring an enterprise knowledge graph for investment analysis. In: Groth, P., et al. (eds.) ISWC 2016. LNCS, vol. 9982, pp. 418–436. Springer, Cham (2016). https://doi.org/10.1007/978-3-319-46547-0_35
26. Liu, J., Lu, Z., Du, W.: Combining enterprise knowledge graph and news sentiment analysis for stock price prediction. In: Proceedings of the 52nd Hawaii International Conference on System Sciences (2019)
27. Gerber, D., Hellmann, S., Bühmann, L., Soru, T., Usbeck, R., Ngonga Ngomo, A.-C.: Real-time RDF extraction from unstructured data streams. In: Alani, H., et al. (eds.) ISWC 2013. LNCS, vol. 8218, pp. 135–150. Springer, Heidelberg (2013). https://doi.org/10.1007/978-3-642-41335-3_9
28. Yahya, M., et al.: Natural language questions for the web of data. In: Proceedings of the 2012 Joint Conference on Empirical Methods in Natural Language Processing and Computational Natural Language Learning, Jeju Island, Korea, pp. 379–390. Association for Computational Linguistics (2012)
29. Shi, B., Weninger, T.: ProjE: embedding projection for knowledge graph completion. In: Thirty-First AAAI Conference on Artificial Intelligence (2017)
30. Bhatia, S., Vishwakarma, H.: Know thy neighbors, and more!: studying the role of context in entity recommendation. In: Proceedings of the 29th on Hypertext and Social Media. ACM (2018)
31. Luconi, F.L., Malone, T.W., Morton, M.S.S.: Expert systems: the next challenge for managers. Sloan Manag. Rev. **27**(4), 3–14 (1986)
32. Wang, Q., et al.: Knowledge graph embedding: a survey of approaches and applications. IEEE Trans. Knowl. Data Eng. **29**(12), 2724–2743 (2017)
33. Shi, L., et al., Semantic health knowledge graph: semantic integration of heterogeneous medical knowledge and services. BioMed Res. Int. **2017**(4), 1–12 (2017)

Reducing Consultant Information Asymmetry in Enterprise System Implementation Projects - The Transaction Cost Economics View

Przemysław Lech[(⊠)]

Faculty of Management, University of Gdańsk,
81-704 Sopot Armii Krajowej 101, Gdańsk, Poland
Przemyslaw.lech@ug.edu.pl

Abstract. This study presents the results of a case study on the level of involvement needed to reduce the information asymmetry with regards to the scope of the Enterprise System implementation. The results show that the cost of determining the particulars of the transaction are too high for the parties to bear before the transaction is actually carried out. The hold-up problem, therefore, exists, as proposed by the Transaction Cost Economics.

Keywords: Consulting · ERP · Project management · Contracting · Scope determination

1 Introduction

Enterprise Systems (ES) have been studied for at least two decades from many angles. Many of this research concentrated on the determination of the success factors, which increase the probability of the project success and on the system acceptance criteria from different stakeholders. However, not much research has been made up-to-date with regards to the phenomena of information and knowledge asymmetry between the parties involved in the Enterprise System implementation project. This paper presents the results of the preliminary study on the level of involvement needed to reduce the information asymmetry with regards to the project scope. The paper is structured as follows. First, a review of the theories involved is presented. Information asymmetry, Agency Theory and Transaction Cost economics are briefly described. Then, the results of a single case study are presented. The study aimed to determine the level of involvement, both from the consulting company and the client, which is needed to determine the scope of the project with a high level of confidence.

2 Review of the Theories

2.1 Information Asymmetry and Agency Theory

Information asymmetry is the situation when one party of a transaction possesses better information than the other party or parties, which puts her in a potentially favourable

© Springer Nature Switzerland AG 2019
S. Wrycza and J. Maślankowski (Eds.): SIGSAND/PLAIS 2019, LNBIP 359, pp. 12–19, 2019.
https://doi.org/10.1007/978-3-030-29608-7_2

situation (Clarkson et al. 2007). The party with better information may tend to behave opportunistically. Opportunistic behaviour is defined as self-interest seeking with guile (Dawson et al. 2010).

The possible ways of reducing information asymmetry are signalling (Spence 1973; Connelly et al. 2011) and screening (Stiglitz 1975). Signalling is an action performed by a better-informed party in which this party communicates the information about the quality of a good to be traded, usually in an indirect way. Screening is an action performed by the under informed party, in which he/she obtains the hidden information or induces the other party to reveal it. In the classical Information Asymmetry theory, information is treated as a commodity, which can be purchased or acquired otherwise at a given price/cost, and the information asymmetry can thus be reduced. Haines and Goodhue (2003) also point out that in some situations, the parties may want to reveal the hidden information at no cost. Although the problem of information asymmetry was initially investigated with regards to spot trades, like car sales, it also affects long-term relationships, as projects. In this second case, information asymmetry is tightly correlated with Agency Theory. An **agency relationship** is "a contract under which one or more persons, the principal(s), engage another person, the agent, to perform some service on their behalf that involves delegating some decision-making authority to the agent. If both parties to the relationship are utility maximizers, there is good reason to believe that the agent will not always act in the best interests of the principal" (Jensen and Meckling 1976), and s/he may behave opportunistically. As the principal typically does not have full information about the agent's behaviour and goals, much of agency theory focuses on designing the appropriate control strategies. The two basic control strategies are behaviour-based (monitoring) and outcome-based (metering) (Haines and Goodhue 2003). Monitoring means keeping track of the agent's behaviour systematically in order to collect information about it (Mahaney and Lederer 2010). The principal "invests in an information source (such as a supervisor) to oversee the agent. Monitoring assumes that the principal can, within a reasonable price, obtain sufficient information to reduce agent opportunism" (Dawson et al. 2010). Metering means evaluating an outcome of the agent's activities and comparing the actual outcome with the one expected by the principal (Dawson et al. 2010).

Both Information Asymmetry and Agency Theory assume that possessing private information, not available to the other party would lead to opportunistic behaviour of the better-informed party.

2.2 Transaction Cost Economics

Transaction Cost Economics (TCE) states that there are transaction costs related to every governance structure, and their level depends on the following attributes of the transaction: uncertainty, the frequency with which transaction occurs, and the level of transaction-specific investments/asset specificity (Williamson 1981). Out of those three attributes, the transaction-specific investment/asset specificity needs explanation. The transaction specific investment takes place when specific assets have to be created to execute the transaction. Such specific assets cannot be easily redeployed to alternative uses without significant loss of productive value (Williamson 1991). Asset specificity is commonly related to the production and trade of highly idiosyncratic goods. i.e. goods which cannot be easily traded elsewhere. Once an investment into specific assets has been made, buyer and seller are effectively operating in a bilateral (or at least quasi-bilateral) exchange relation for a considerable period.

The agents should choose the governance structure, which minimises the sum of the transaction costs and production costs. The transaction cost economics predicts that transactions which differ in their attributes are aligned with governance structures, which differ in their abilities to adapt to disturbances, coordinating mechanisms, incentive level, and control mechanisms (Williamson 1991). There are three types of governance structures to choose from: market, hierarchy and hybrid. Market governance is characterised by the autonomous adaptation to disturbances, no coordination mechanisms (except the market price mechanism), and limited administrative control (limited to courts). Hierarchy allows for coordinated and gradual adaptation to disturbances and involves strong coordination mechanisms and strong administrative control (authority relation).

Hybrid governance structures lie in the middle. Hybrid is a governance structure, in which the autonomy of the parties is preserved, but there is a bilateral dependency between the parties due to the transaction-specific investments. The parties are realising their own, separate agendas, and have separate profit streams, as on the classical market. On the other hand, due to the non-trivial level of the transaction-specific investment, which will be lost if the transaction is terminated, they are interested in continuing the relationship, the so-called hold-up problem. The most frequently mentioned form of hybrid governance is long term contracting of a different kind (Ménard 2004; Williamson 2008). Hybrid governance allows both for autonomous and coordinated adaptation to disturbances, but at a higher cost compared to market and hierarchy respectively. This is because autonomous adaptation is related to the possible loss of transaction-specific investments, and coordinated adaptation requires bilateral arrangements between autonomous parties (cannot be achieved by fiat, as in hierarchy). The control has to be performed via monitoring and metering and requires additional governance mechanisms from the principal, which also come at a non-trivial cost.

3 Characteristics of an Enterprise System Implementation Project

Enterprise System is a standard, configurable, and customizable, multi-component application suite that includes integrated business solutions for the major business processes and the management functions of an enterprise. It typically includes both transactional and analytical applications, such as Enterprise Resource Planning, Customer Relationship Management, Supply Chain Management, Content Management, Business Intelligence/Business Analytics and others, and constitutes the primary source of management information and the main tool for managing business processes in an enterprise (Lech 2019).

Implementation of an Enterprise System in a company is a complex project which affects most of the core business processes and requires high involvement from a large number of business stakeholders (Lech 2019). It requires highly specialised, knowledge regarding the system functionality, as well as project management and governance capabilities, which is difficult and costly to acquire in-house (Lech 2014). Therefore such projects are commonly executed in cooperation with a specialised consulting company, and a hybrid governance structure is in place.

This situation poses implications outlined by the Information Asymmetry and Agency Theories. Mahaney and Lederer (2003) provided a research framework for examining Information Systems projects with the use of Agency Theory. Turner and Müller (2004) explored communication between the agent and the principal as the key factor for decreasing the probability of opportunistic behaviour. Dawson et al. (2010) found out that two-sided information asymmetry in Information Systems projects may lead both consultants and clients to behave opportunistically. They also suggested that the level of information asymmetry, together with explicit and tacit knowledge needed to reduce it, makes it challenging to construct a formal contract between the parties. Haines and Goodhue (2003) suggest that the higher level of Information System knowledge of the client limits the possibility of the consultants to behave opportunistically. They indicate that the willingness of the consultants to share their knowledge with the client is crucial to the success of the project. Wachnik (2014) suggests that the client faces problems on every stage of a project due to lack of information regarding the system. Haaskjold et al. (2019) investigate the factors affecting transaction cost and collaboration in the projects of different kind. They find owner's organizational efficiency, project uncertainty, quality of communication and trust as the main factors influencing the collaboration. Kaim et al. (2019) argument that agile project management may be the remedy for reducing the transaction cost in complex IT projects. None of this research concentrated on the information asymmetry of the consulting enterprise (consultant).

This paper aims to examine another aspect related to the information asymmetry, i.e. what level of involvement both from the client and the consultant is necessary to reduce the information asymmetry of the consultant to determine the project scope in such a way that a non-trivial contract can be signed between the parties. The answer to this question would indicate the level of transaction-specific investments from the consultant and the client necessary to reduce the scope of uncertainty in the contract.

4 Research Design

The research is based on a single case-study design (Yin 2009). The unit of analysis was a full-scope, greenfield SAP ECC (Enterprise Resource Planning Central Component) project in a medium-sized production company. The project involved five functional areas (financial accounting, controlling, purchasing and warehouse management, sales and distribution, production planning and execution), and lasted for fifteen months. The data collection methods included longitudinal participant observation and analysis of the consultants' reports, in which they reported the performed activities, together with the workload. The study aimed at answering the following research question:

RQ: What level of involvement both from the client and the consultant is necessary to reduce the information asymmetry of the consultant to determine the project scope?

5 Research Results

The consultants were asked, at what stage of the project, they are able to determine the scope of the implementation in their respective functional areas with a high level of confidence. All five consultants answered that this is possible after the Business Blueprint phase of the project. Business Blueprint phase is one of the initial phases of the SAP system implementation project, which consists of the analytical and design steps, and which ends up with the preparation of the so-called Blueprint document, including:

- Description of the client business processes which are subject to implementation (with the use of a business process notation – usually Business Process Model and Notation – BPMN or Event-Driven Process Chain – EPC, and in natural language);
- A high-level description of non-process related requirements (RICEF – Reports, Interfaces, Conversions, Extensions, Forms);
- A high-level description of how the processes and requirements will be executed in the future Enterprise System, i.e. how the system will be configured and if needed, customised to meet the requirements.

The Blueprint document is subject to review and approval by the client and is a base for further configuration and customisation of the system.

Therefore, the work performed during the Blueprint phase of the project was analysed further. According to the activity reports, submitted by the consultants, the workload in the Business Blueprint phase involved 157.5 consulting days, which constituted 32% of the total project workload. Out of those 157.5 days, 72.5 days (46%) were dedicated to the workshops with the process owners of the client. Time spent by the client staff to prepare for the workshops, deliver information to the consultants otherwise than during the workshops, and review the documentation was not captured. During the workshops, the functional teams consisting of the consultants and process owners discuss in detail the business processes in their respective areas. If possible, the solutions available in the system to cover those processes were presented. If the process in its current form could not be modelled in the system, alternative solutions were proposed, and either agreed by the team or escalated to the project management. Each workshop resulted in the meeting minutes, which were subject to approval by the client, and were later consolidated into the Business Blueprint document. It is important to notice, that when the client representatives were asked after the project closure if they understood the proposed solutions when approving the Business Blueprint, the answer was "no". Therefore, the information asymmetry was reduced on the consultant side, but it was not the case for the client. The rest of the workload (85 consulting days/54%) during the Business Blueprint phase was dedicated by the consultants to prepare the business process maps, design the respective solutions in the system, and describe them in the Blueprint document. The Business Blueprint phase resulted in 508 pages of documentation (101,6 page per functional area).

Even if one takes into account only the 72,5 days spent by the client and consultant representatives during the workshops, it constitutes 14,5% of the total project workload. The workload from the process owners to prepare additional information, and from the consultants to document the requirements has to be added to this amount, although it was not possible to capture it from the existing documentation. This workload constitutes transaction-specific investment for both parties. If the project is not continued, this investment would be completely lost by the consulting company, as the Blueprint is client-specific and is not transferable in any way to other clients. It will also be at least partially lost by the client. Some of the knowledge, captured during the workshop by the consultants is not easily codified. It remains as tacit knowledge in the heads of the consultants. In other words, if another consulting company was supposed to perform system configuration and customisation basing only on the written Blueprint, it would be hard to achieve. Additional workshops would have to be performed to clarify open issues. To sum up:

1. The workload (and cost) needed to clarify the scope of the project is so high that:
   a. the consulting company would not be willing to perform it free of charge,
   b. the client company would not be willing to perform it several times with different consultants.
2. Therefore, both client and consultant are "locked into" the transaction before the detailed scope, budget and schedule can be determined.

This leads to an interesting paradox: **the cost of determining the particulars of the transaction are too high for the parties to bear before the transaction is actually carried out.**

The above conclusion is in line with the predictions from the Transaction Cost Economics. The hold-up problem exists in Enterprise System implementations in its extreme form.

To deal with this paradox the parties may sign the 'null' or 'frame' contract on a time and materials basis. The consultants are then being paid according to their actual workload. The client has to implement monitoring mechanisms to control the consultants and impose strong discipline on its own staff to manage the scope. Another way is to sign the fixed-price contract before the Blueprint is known, basing on incomplete information. Such an approach poses a high risk of future contract re-negotiation, once the details of the scope are revealed.

6 Conclusions

This paper examined the involvement of the client and the consultant, necessary to reduce the information asymmetry of the consultant with regards to the scope of an Enterprise system implementation project. The study revealed, that the workload from consultants to determine the scope falls between 14,5 and 32% of the total project workload. Similar involvement is required from the client. This constitutes a transaction-specific investment, which will be lost if the contract is terminated. The level of this investment is high enough to make the parties locked-into the transaction before the actual details this transaction are known. The implications of this fact for the client are that classical approaches to selecting a trade partner, bidding and contracting are not feasible for Enterprise System implementations. Alternative approaches, including screening, getting opinions from other companies, reference visits should be applied for implementation partner selection. As the determination of the project scope in detail is too costly before signing the contract, time and materials approach, with tight scope management and monitoring mechanisms is the preferred solution.

7 Limitations of the Study and Future Research

The main limitation of this study is related to the fact, that it was based on a single case. The amount of involvement, needed reduce the information asymmetry may differ in other cases due to such factors as experience of the consultants from previous projects in a similar industries, experience of the client with using similar technology, availability of pre-configured demo scenarios in the system, eagerness of the client to adjust business to the system standard, and others. This needs further research. Another direction of future research is related to the ways in which organisations deal with Enterprise System project contracting, how they overcome the hold-up problem, and what governance mechanisms should be used to successfully deliver a project. The latter research problem was discussed in relation to other types of projects. The research shows the role of relationship-based procurement methods, such as partnering, integrated project delivery and alliancing (Haaskjold et al. 2019; Walker and Lloyd-Walker 2015). It also highlights relational contracting, involving long-term commitment, trust, communication and collaboration as a way to reduce transaction costs in projects (Benítez-Ávila et al. 2018; Chakkol et al. 2018). These aspects should be further investigated in relation to the IT projects involving external contractors.

References

Benítez-Ávila, C., Hartmann, A., Dewulf, G., Henseler, J.: Interplay of relational and contractual governance in public-private partnerships: the mediating role of relational norms, trust and partners' contribution. Int. J. Project Manag. 36(3), 429–443 (2018)

Chakkol, M., Selviaridis, K., Finne, M.: The governance of collaboration in complex projects. Int. J. Oper. Prod. Manag. 38(4), 997–1019 (2018)

Clarkson, G., Jacobsen, T.E., Batcheller, A.L.: Information asymmetry and information sharing. Gov. Inf. Q. 24(4), 827–839 (2007)

Connelly, B.L., Certo, S.T., Ireland, R.D., Reutzel, C.R.: Signaling theory: a review and assessment. J. Manag. 37(1), 39–67 (2011)

Dawson, G.S., Watson, R.T., Boudreau, M.-C.: Information asymmetry in information systems consulting: toward a theory of relationship constraints. J. Manag. Inf. Syst. 27(3), 143–177 (2010)

Haaskjold, H., Andersen, B., Lædre, O., Aarseth, W.: Factors affecting transaction costs and collaboration in projects. Int. J. Manag. Projects Bus. (2019)

Haines, M.N., Goodhue, D.L.: Implementation partner involvement and knowledge transfer in the context of ERP implementations. Int. J. Hum.-Comput. Interact. 16(1), 23–38 (2003)

Jensen, M., Meckling, W.: Theory of the firm: managerial behavior, agency costs, and ownership structure. J. Finan. Econ. 3(4), 305–360 (1976)

Kaim, R., Härting, R.-C., Reichstein, C.: Benefits of agile project management in an environment of increasing complexity—a transaction cost analysis. In: Czarnowski, I., Howlett, R.J., Jain,

L.C. (eds.) Intelligent Decision Technologies 2019. SIST, vol. 143, pp. 195–204. Springer, Singapore (2019). https://doi.org/10.1007/978-981-13-8303-8_17

Lech, P.: Managing knowledge in IT projects: a framework for enterprise system implementation. J. Knowl. Manag. **18**(3), 551–573 (2014)

Lech, P.: Enterprise system implementations in transition and developed economies: differences in project contracting and governance. Inf. Technol. Dev. **25**(2), 357–380 (2019)

Mahaney, R.C., Lederer, A.L.: Information systems project management: an agency theory interpretation. J. Syst. Softw. **68**(1), 1–9 (2003)

Ménard, C.: The economics of hybrid organizations. J. Inst. Theor. Econ. **160**(3), 345–376 (2004)

Spence, M.: Job market signaling. Q. J. Econ. **87**(3), 355–374 (1973)

Stiglitz, J.E.: The theory the of "screening " education, and the distribution of income. Am. Econ. Rev. **65**(3), 283–300 (1975)

Turner, J.R., Müller, R.: Communication and co-operation on projects between the project owner as principal and the project manager as agent. Eur. Manag. J. **22**(3), 327–336 (2004)

Wachnik, B.: Reducing information asymmetry in IT projects. Informatyka Ekonomiczna **1**(31), 212–222 (2014)

Walker, D., Lloyd-Walker, B.M.: Collaborative Project Procurement Arrangements. Project Management Institute, Newton Square (2015)

Williamson, O.E.: The economics of organization: the transaction cost approach. Am. J. Sociol. **87**(3), 548–577 (1981)

Williamson, O.E.: Comparative economic organization: the analysis of discrete structural alternatives. Adm. Sci. Q. **36**(2), 269–296 (1991)

Williamson, O.E.: Outsourcing: transaction cost economics and supply chain management. J. Supply Chain Manag. Glob. Rev. Purch. Supply **44**(2), 5–16 (2008)

Yin, R.: Case Study Research Design and Methods, 4th edn. Sage, Thousand Oaks (2009)

A Study of the Impact of Internal and External Usability on Knowledge Transfer by the Means of Mobile Technologies: Preliminary Results

Paweł Weichbroth[1] [ID] and Michał Kuciapski[2(✉)] [ID]

[1] WSB University in Gdańsk, Grunwaldzka 238A, 80-266 Gdańsk, Poland
`pweichbroth@wsb.gda.pl`
[2] University of Gdańsk, Jana Bażyńskiego 8, 80-309 Gdańsk, Poland
`m.kuciapski@ug.edu.pl`

Abstract. In this paper, we raise a discussion on the results of an empirical study of the impact of internal and external usability on knowledge transfer by the means of mobile technologies. Firstly, based on an extensive literature review and analysis, we have identified both technology acceptance and usability models with their associated variables, along with their definitions. Secondly, having formulated inclusion (exclusion) criteria, we have selected 10 variables, namely perceived enjoyment, activities availability, system accessibility, cognitive load, performance expectancy, user autonomy, relative usability, learnability, memorability and facilitating conditions. In general, this set constitutes both upper-level internal and external usability variables. To collect data we have used the survey instrument, which in a pilot study was successfully submitted to 70 employees who declared themselves to be advanced users of mobile devices, applications and services. The results of the statistical analysis show that only external usability impacts the intention by employees to use mobile technologies for knowledge transfer. On the other hand, being an external variable, it also has an impact on internal usability, which means that the perceived usability of mobile applications directly depends on the perceived usability of mobile devices, in particular, the perceived performance of the installed operating system.

Keywords: Internal usability · External usability · Technology acceptance · Knowledge transfer · Mobile technologies · Employees

1 Introduction

In the area of the knowledge-based economy, knowledge transfer matters more than ever. By its nature, this process is intangible and human-intensive. However, the adoption of information communication technologies (ICTs) has changed the facets of the phenomenon completely. The limitations and obstacles related to the psychical form of knowledge capacity and storage, mobility and availability, have been decisively eliminated. Nevertheless, other issues have emerged concerning users' attitudes toward technology acceptance.

© Springer Nature Switzerland AG 2019
S. Wrycza and J. Maślankowski (Eds.): SIGSAND/PLAIS 2019, LNBIP 359, pp. 20–33, 2019.
https://doi.org/10.1007/978-3-030-29608-7_3

The Technology Acceptance Model (TAM) [1], which is widely used to investigate user adoption and acceptance of new technologies and systems, is influenced by two internal factors: perceived usefulness (PU) and perceived ease of use (PEOU). The former is "the degree to which a person believes that using a particular system would enhance his or her job performance", while the latter is "the degree to which a person believes that using a particular system would be free of effort" [2]. Two other factors are attitude toward use (A) and behavioral intention to use (BI).

PU and PEOU are affected by external variables, such as management support, participation in training, tool functionality, task characteristics, prior similar experience and relevant skills [3]. The former focuses on the benefits of technology and therefore is considered to be a variable that is related to use [4], while the latter is associated with users' evaluation of the effort involved in the improvement of using the technology [5]. In general terms, the relationship between them can be defined as a cause-and-effect rule (PEOU → PU), while in detail, the believed effort to engage is the premise, and the believed benefits to be obtained is the conclusion.

In recent years, a large body of literature has documented attempts to develop alternate learning technologies for computer-aided learning. The emergence of wireless networking technologies and a variety of mobile-device innovations have received a great deal of attention in the field of knowledge management [6]. The features of mobile devices, such as context sensitivity, portability, social connectivity, are just a few reasons for the shift from desktop computers [7, 8]. Mobile devices have made knowledge transfer movable, collaborative, gamified, real-time and omnipresent [9, 10]. However, they have certain limitations due to the hardware layer (bandwidth, display size, peripherals, storage capacity) and the software layer (functionality, single window, user interaction). As a result, usability, measured by efficiency, effectiveness, learnability and user satisfaction, suffers from these properties and obstacles [11, 12]. In this paper, we introduce a framework which grounds the theory of the impact of internal and external usability on knowledge transfer, performed by the means of mobile technologies. To the best of our knowledge, no study of Human-Computer Interaction (HCI) or information systems (IS) has comprehensively examined internal and external usability variables in mobile settings. The findings of this research have theoretical implications for mobile usability research and practical implications for mobile user experience design.

The study of the subject matter literature pointed out the existence of many variables connected with technology usability, of which a few have very convergent meanings. As a result, the theoretical framework includes ten of them. Exemplary assertion statements for the variables proved that all of them have an internal and external usability perspective and are probably interrelated. Therefore, the final model assumes that external usability and internal usability directly impact technology acceptance, and external usability influences internal usability.

The rest of the paper is organized as follows. In the second section, the related research is discussed, in which usability variables are depicted and identified in existing models. The third section presents the proposed research model and three stated research hypotheses. The penultimate section points out future research directions. The article finishes with conclusions.

2 Related Research

Usability has been a major subject matter in human–computer interaction (HCI) research. In spite of the apparent ambiguity regarding the definition of usability, typically it has been simply associated with the notion of the ease of using a target object, and ultimately the achieved satisfaction by its user. In general terms, widely recognized and accepted is the definition provided by the ISO Organization, where usability is the "degree to which a product or system can be used by specified users to achieve specified goals with effectiveness, efficiency and satisfaction in a specified context of use; it can either be specified or measured as a product quality characteristic in terms of its sub-characteristics, or specified or measured directly by measures that are a subset of quality in use" [13]. In a more narrow sense, usability is the "extent to which a product can be used by specified users to achieve specified goals with effectiveness, efficiency and satisfaction in a specified context of use" [14].

The reference search procedure proposed by Cooper [15] was used to collect relevant usability and technology acceptance references. Electronic searches and manual reference list retrieval were used to collect valid data, ensuring data only written in English. The major databases used for the electronic searches were Elsevier, IEEE, Springer, and Web of Science. Based on the key model and key words in the previous research of technology acceptance models [16, 17], knowledge management [18, 19] and mobile usability [20], the three following sets of key words, and combinations thereof, were used to construct queries executed against specified scientific databases: (1) TAM, technology acceptance model, technology acceptance, perceived ease of use, perceived usefulness, (2) knowledge management | transfer, education, teaching, training, learning, and (3) usability, mobile usability | device | technology, portable. The three sets of keywords were integrated systematically with Boolean operators, using the "OR" operator within the set and the "AND" operator between the sets. The manual reference list retrieval was performed only for full-text papers, after reviewing their abstracts. In summary, to amass the gathered qualitative data in the study subject, another round of searches was conducted again using the extracted reference lists to find any neglected but relevant work.

In accordance with the presented research method, Table 1 presents the set of 19 identified usability variables and corresponding models which served as a foundation to construct the theory of the usability framework for knowledge transfer facilitated by mobile technologies.

Table 1. Usability variables with definitions and corresponding models.

Publication	Basic model	Usability variable	Variable definition (explanation)
[21]	Activity theory	System satisfaction (SS)	Enjoyment of using the system for retrieving and gathering online content
		System activities (SA)	Convenience of using the system for reading and retrieving online content
		System functions (SF)	Ease of using the system for gathering and retrieving online content
[22]	TAM, Social motivational theory	System accessibility (SAC)	Ease of getting and accessing information (content); compatibility with other computer devices
[23]	Theory of planned behavior (TPB)	Perceived self-efficacy (PSE)	Confidence and comfort of using a device
[24]	TAM	Satisfaction (S)	Perceived benefits and fulfilled expectations of using a device (external) and system (internal)
		Perceived control & skill (PCS)	Justified belief in a device and the system control and manipulation
[17]	Unified theory of acceptance and use of technology (UTAUT)	Relative usability (RU)	Effort expectancy and performance expectancy to use a given technology in relation to other solutions
		User autonomy (UA)	Perceived autonomy and flexibility in technology use
[25]	TAM	Learnability (L)	Perceived efficiency and ease in learning the application
		Memorability (M)	Perceived understanding of the application capabilities Ability to recreate the understanding of the application capabilities over time
[26]	TAM	Perceived enjoyment (PE)	Intrinsic motivation that emphasizes the usage process and reflects the pleasure and enjoyment associated with using a system
[27]	TAM, Theory of reasoned action (TRA), UTAUT	Perceived usefulness (PU)	Belief in the improvement and progress of self-performance through using a technology
[28]	Theory of organizational information services (TOIS), UTAUT	Self-efficacy (SE)	Personal judgement to use a technology to accomplish a given job or task

(continued)

Table 1. (*continued*)

Publication	Basic model	Usability variable	Variable definition (explanation)
[29]	UTAUT	Computer self-efficacy (CSE)	Personal self-evaluated ability to use a technology to accomplish a reflected job or task
[30–33]	UTAUT	Facilitating conditions (FC)	"The degree to which an individual believes that an organizational and technical infrastructure exists to support the use of the system"
		Effort expectancy (EE)	"The degree of ease associated with the use of the system"
		Performance expectancy (PE)	"The degree to which an individual believes that using the system will help him or her to attain gains in job performance"
[33]	Cognitive Load Theory (CLT)	Cognitive load (CL)	Internal: "the difficulty level of the instructional content, resulting from the amount of inter-correlation between essential elements in the instructional material" External: "the unnecessary load imposed by poorly designed instruction" Germane: "the mental effort that is consciously invested by learners while processing elements of the internal load"

According to the results of the performed literature study, some variable definitions were not defined accurately and in a few cases were not even provided. The analysis and synthesis, applied to both the internal and external usability facets of the knowledge transfer, enabled us to formulate adequate definitions which encompass the context-specific setting of the usage of mobile technologies for knowledge transfer (Table 1).

Technology acceptance variables connected with usability exist in many proposals based on theories or models regarding technology acceptance: Activity theory, Social motivational theory, Theory of planned behaviour, Theory of organizational information services, Theory of reasoned action, Technology acceptance model and Unified theory of acceptance and use of technology (Table 1). Moreover, the subject matter analysis points out that new variables explaining technology acceptance connected with the usability of applications and devices have been positively verified over a significant time since 2003.

3 Research Methodology

3.1 Research Model and Hypotheses

Study of the subject matter literature presented in the second section of the article, also included in previously conducted research (authors), highlighted the existence of many variables related to the usability of mobile technologies. Some of them have convergent meanings with others. In such a situation, it was assumed that the model will omit variables (Table 2):

- with a more narrow meaning,
- subjective or context-specific by design, and as a consequence, rarely referenced.

Table 2. Omitted variables.

Omitted variable	Convergent variable	Omission reason
System satisfaction (SS)	Perceived enjoyment (PEJ)	Less general character
System activities (SA)	Activities availability (AA)	Less presented in the subject matter literature
Perceived control & skill (PCS) effort expectancy (EE)	Cognitive load (CL)	More narrow meaning
Perceived self-efficacy (PSE) self-efficacy (SE)	Performance expectancy (PE)	Less general character

Seven variables were omitted (Table 2). As a result, the research model integrated the following technology acceptance determinants:

- perceived enjoyment (PEJ) in [26],
- activities availability (AA) in [21],
- system accessibility (SAC) in [22],
- cognitive load (CL) in [33],
- performance expectancy (PE) in [30],
- user autonomy (UA) in [17],
- relative usability (RU) in [17],
- learnability (L) in [25],
- memorability (M) in [25],
- facilitating conditions (FC) in [30].

As the aim of the article was to propose a model explaining the internal and external usability impact on technology acceptance, the variables were grouped as internal and external ones, where:

- internal perspective concerns the usability of the application;
- external perspective is connected with the usability of the environment used by the application, understood as the device and operating system.

To decide which variables are appropriate to measure the influence of internal and external technology usability on the intention to use it, exemplary assertion statements were prepared (Table 3).

Table 3. Exemplary assertion statements for the internal and external usability context of variables.

Variable	Assertion statement	
	Internal	External
PEJ	I enjoy utilizing mobile applications	I enjoy utilizing mobile devices and their operating systems
AA	Mobile applications allow activities to be realized in a convenient way	Mobile devices and their operating systems allow activities to be realized in a convenient way
SAC	Access to resources with the use of mobile applications is easy	Access to resources with the use of mobile devices and their operating systems is easy
CL	When using mobile applications it is possible to conduct other activities	When using mobile devices and their operating systems it is possible to conduct other activities
PE	The use of mobile applications increases efficiency in the realization of activities	The use of mobile devices and their operating systems increases efficiency in the realization of activities
UA	Mobile applications allow activities to be conducted in a more individual way	Mobile devices and their operating systems allow for conducting activities in an individual way
RU	The use of mobile applications is at least as convenient as with alternative solutions (e.g. desktop)	The use of mobile devices and their operating systems is at least as convenient as with alternative solutions (e.g. desktop)
L	Learning how to use mobile applications is fast and easy	Learning how to use mobile devices and their operating systems is fast and easy
M	Even after a long time it is still possible to use mobile applications efficiently	Even after a long time it is still possible to use mobile devices and their operating systems efficiently
FC	Mobile applications are an easy solution to implement	Mobile devices and their operating systems allow for convenient use of mobile applications

Table 3 highlights that all variables have logical assertion statements, both from the internal and external usability perspective. Therefore both groups – internal usability and external usability – contain all variables. As particular variables have been confirmed by researchers to directly impact the intention to use technology (Table 3), the elaborated model includes connections between internal and external groups of variables and dependent variables (Fig. 1). It seems likely that environments of using applications related to the devices and operating systems used influence the perceived usability of applications. Therefore, the connection between external usability and internal usability is an integral part of the proposed model (Fig. 1).

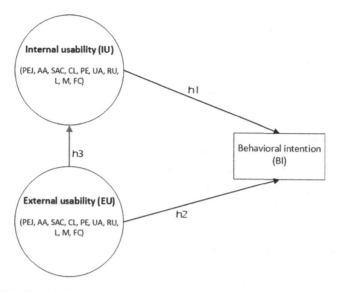

Fig. 1. Model of the internal and external usability impact on technology acceptance.

According to Fig. 1, the assumed relationships between grouped variables will be verified by the stated hypotheses presented in Table 4.

Table 4. Research hypotheses.

Hypoth. no.	Connection	Description
H1	IU → BI	Internal usability directly influences the intention to use mobile technologies
H2	EU → BI	External usability directly influences the intention to use mobile technologies
H3	EU → IU	External usability directly influences the perceived internal usability of mobile technologies

The validation methodology of the proposed model, based on the verification of stated hypotheses (Table 4) is presented in the following Subsect. 3.2.

3.2   Model Validation Methodology

The validation of the stated hypothesis and therefore the proposed model was based on a survey among users of mobile technologies. The questionnaire began with an explanation of key concepts, such as: m-learning, mobile devices, knowledge transfer, internal and external usability. The crucial part of the survey included 71 statement assertions formulated in accordance with acceptance questionnaire rules, while also taking into account m-learning and the competence development context – 3–5 statements for each variable. Each question was measured using a 7-point Likert scale. The assertion statements in the survey were created for all variables included in the elaborated model (Fig. 1).

During the pilot study the research data was collected via a CAWI survey during face-to-face meetings. Because of the lack of a reliable sampling frame, it is difficult to conduct random sampling for all potential mobile technology users. Similar to Wang et al. [34], this study adopted a non-random sampling technique (i.e. convenience sampling) to start collecting the sample data. To be able to generalize the results, the survey data was later collected with a snowball sampling technique, from many organizations in Poland, from both the public and private sectors and with a diverse number of employees. As a result, the survey was conducted among 70 employees, whom all knew how to use mobile devices, applications and services, and were able to report on their experience. The data was collected in a 3-month period, starting from January 2019.

Structural equation modelling (SEM) was utilized for data collected via the survey to validate the model. SEM has been widely tested in the field of technology acceptance. The advantage of SEM is that it considers both the evaluation of the measurement model and the estimation of the structural coefficient at the same time. A two-step modelling approach, recommended by Anderson and Gerbing [35], as well as McDonald and Ho [36], was followed in such a way that the confirmatory factor analysis (CFA) was carried out first to provide an assessment of convergent and discriminant validity. Inter-construct correlation coefficient estimates were examined along with a particular item's internal consistency reliability, by using Cronbach's alpha coefficient estimates [37]. The model quality was measured with key CFA fit indices, such as:

- $\chi 2$/d.f.,
- GFI (Goodness of Fit Index),
- CFI (Comparative Fit Index),
- RMSEA (Root Mean Square Error of Approximation).

As CFA fit indices had values within the recommended range, stated hypotheses were verified through a regression analysis with SEM through significance levels and standardized β-coefficients.

4   Research Results

A data validity test was performed to reduce the possibility of receiving incorrect answers during the data collection period [38], which showed that all questionnaires were valid. The inter-construct correlation coefficient estimates were examined along with a particular item's internal consistency by using Cronbach's alpha coefficient estimates (Table 5).

Table 5. Data reliability.

Variable	Cronbach's alpha	Cronbach's alpha based on standardized items
IU	0.972	0.972
EU	0.983	0.984
BI	0.952	0.952

Reliability values greater than 0.7 are considered as acceptable [39]. All items far exceeded the recommended level. As a result, the data was internally consistent and acceptable, with a total reliability equal to 0.989.

Values of model fit indices checked via CFA, which is an integral part of SEM, are presented in Table 6.

Table 6. Fit indices of the model.

Fit indices	Recommended value	Result
χ^2/d.f.	<3	2.083
GFI (Goodness of fit index)	>0.8	0.812
CFI (Comparative fit index)	>0.9	0.974
RMSEA (Root mean square error of approximation)	<0.08	0.076

Four fit indices satisfied by the elaborated model (Table 6) confirm its validity and, through a regression analysis, enable the three stated hypotheses given in Table 4 and included in Fig. 1 to be verified. The verification results of the research hypotheses are contained in Table 7.

Table 7. Research hypotheses verification.

Hypoth. number	Connection	Significance (p)	Standardized β-coefficient	Verification result
H1	IU → BI	0.295	0.264	Rejected
H2	EU → BI	0.029	0.556	Accepted
H3	EU → IU	<0.001	0.957	Accepted

According to Table 7, two of the three hypotheses were positively verified. The implications are discussed in the following section.

5 Discussion

5.1 Theoretical Implications

Interpreting the theoretical aspects at the outset, external usability (EU) occurred to be the only technology acceptance factor from the usability perspective, hence the second hypothesis (H2) was confirmed in contrast to the first one (H1), as presented in Table 7 and Fig. 2.

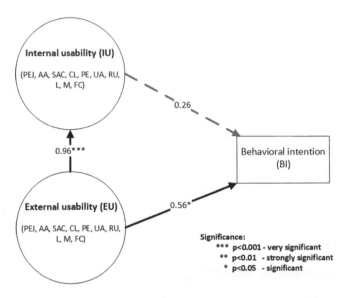

Fig. 2. Technology acceptance model from the internal and external usability perspectives – verification results

The impact of EU on BI was very significant as the p-value was below 0.001 (Fig. 2). The strength of the influence of EU on BI is high ($\beta = 0.556$). This means that employees expect high usability of the mobile environment, understood as a device and its operating system, used during knowledge transfer processes. Surprisingly, internal usability (IU) occurred not to impact the intention of employees to use mobile technologies for knowledge transfer (H1), hence the p-value was higher than the 0.05 reference value (Table 7). This means that the usability of the mobile environment, not the mobile applications used by employees, during the development of competences is important. The study result explains the market consolidation processes of mobile devices and especially operating systems that occurred during recent years. Despite the same applications being offered on various mobile operating systems, such as: Android, BlackBerry, iOS, Symbian and Windows Mobile, only a few operating systems remained on the market.

EU occurred to be also an external variable, hence its impact on IU (H3) has been confirmed (Table 7). As the p-value is below 0.001 and the beta coefficient is almost 1, the influence of EU on IU is very significant and strong, with a nearly linear correlation. It has to be interpreted that the perceived usability of mobile applications used for knowledge transfer directly depends on the perceived usability of utilized mobile devices and their operating systems. Therefore, the same application might be rated differently depending on the device used, such as: e-book reader, smartphone, tablet or netbook, and its operating system.

5.2   Practical Implications

From the practical perspective, the results of the study indicate that the perceived usability of knowledge transfer heavily depends on external factors, such as mobile device performance. Therefore, software providers, to develop mobile applications, should only select such technologies (platforms, frameworks, programming languages) which are fully compliant with hardware devices. On the other hand, effective knowledge transfer implies new requirements which go beyond the scope of the existing patterns, established for mobile solutions. In particular, the different types of mobile hardware devices have increased the risk of a decrease in the quality of the interaction between a user and an application.

5.3   Study Limitations and Further Research

Like any other, this study has its limitations. Firstly, the pilot group to some extent neglected internal usability, which stands in contrast to the "traditional" logic of software product development. In such case, a second run of the study will encompass a larger number of participants. Secondly, a larger sample will allow us to examine intercorrelations not only between upper-level variables (IU, EU and BI), but also between particular variables.

Further research should be conducted to once again test the impact of internal usability, through a survey tailored to the specifics of technology acceptance and with a proper statistical approach, like structural equation modelling. Measuring significance levels and standardized β-coefficients of paths would allow us to support (reject) internal usability. The results will be an important contribution to the technology acceptance research field, especially in the case of confirmed paths between model variables.

6   Conclusions

The primary outcome of the performed study on the impact of internal and external usability is the statistically confirmed significance of the latter variable, regarding the intention to use mobile technologies to transfer knowledge among employees. Moreover, the research results highlighted that external usability has a very significant and strong influence on internal usability, with nearly a linear correlation. Surprisingly, internal usability occurred not to impact the intention of employees to use mobile technologies for knowledge transfer. This might be related to the number of survey participants during the pilot study as structural equation modelling, used for the proposed model validation, is sensitive in this regard.

References

1. Davis, F.D.: Perceived usefulness, perceived ease of use, and user acceptance of information technology. MIS Q. **13**(3), 318–340 (1989)
2. Davis, F.D., Bagozzi, R.P., Warshaw, P.R.: User acceptance of computer technology: a comparison of two theoretical models. Manag. Sci. **35**(8), 982–1003 (1989)

3. Legris, P., Ingham, J., Collerette, P.: Why do people use information technology? A critical review of the technology acceptance model. Inf. Manag. **40**(3), 191–204 (2003). https://doi.org/10.1016/S0378-7206(01)00143-4

4. Scherer, R., Hatlevik, O.E.: "Sore eyes and distracted" or "excited and confident"? – The role of perceived negative consequences of using ICT for perceived usefulness and self-efficacy. Comput. Educ. **115**, 188–200 (2017). https://doi.org/10.1016/j.compedu.2017.08.003

5. Ozturk, A.B., Bilgihan, A., Nusair, K., Okumus, F.: What keeps the mobile hotel booking users loyal? Investigating the roles of self-efficacy, compatibility, perceived ease of use, and perceived convenience. Int. J. Inf. Manag. **36**(6), 1350–1359 (2016). https://doi.org/10.1016/j.ijinfomgt.2016.04.005

6. Kuciapski, M.: Students acceptance of m-learning for higher education – UTAUT model validation. In: Wrycza, S. (ed.) SIGSAND/PLAIS 2016. LNBIP, vol. 264, pp. 155–166. Springer, Cham (2016). https://doi.org/10.1007/978-3-319-46642-2_11

7. Chinnery, G.M.: Emerging technologies: going to the mall: mobile assisted language learning. Lang. Learn. Technol. **10**(1), 9–16 (2006)

8. Weichbroth, P.: Delivering usability in IT products: empirical lessons from the field. Int. J. Softw. Eng. Knowl. Eng. **28**(7), 1027–1045 (2018). https://doi.org/10.1142/S0218194018500298

9. Kukulska-Hulme, A.: Will mobile learning change language learning? ReCALL **21**(2), 157–165 (2009)

10. Lai, C., Zheng, D.: Self-directed use of mobile devices for language learning beyond the classroom. ReCALL **30**(3), 1–20 (2017). https://doi.org/10.1017/S0958344017000258

11. Redlarski, K., Weichbroth, P.: Hard lessons learned: delivering usability in IT projects. In: Federated Conference on Computer Science and Information Systems (FedCSIS), pp. 1379–1382. IEEE (2016). https://doi.org/10.15439/2016f20

12. Redlarski, K.: The impact of end-user participation in IT projects on product usability. In: Proceedings of the International Conference on Multimedia, Interaction, Design and Innovation (MIDI), pp. 1–8 (2013)

13. ISO/IEC 25010:2011. https://www.iso.org/obp/ui/#iso:std:iso-iec:25010:ed-1:v1:en

14. ISO 9241-11:2018. https://www.iso.org/obp/ui/#iso:std:iso:9241:-11:ed-2:v1:en

15. Cooper, H.: Research Synthesis and Meta-Analysis: A Step-by-Step Approach, vol. 2. Sage publications, Thousand Oaks (2016)

16. Marangunić, N., Granić, A.: Technology acceptance model: a literature review from 1986 to 2013. Univ. Access Inf. Soc. **14**(1), 81–95 (2015)

17. Kuciapski, M.: A model of mobile technologies acceptance for knowledge transfer by employees. J. Knowl. Manag. **21**(5), 1053–1076 (2017)

18. Costa, E., Soares, A.L., de Sousa, J.P.: Information, knowledge and collaboration management in the internationalisation of SMEs: a systematic literature review. Int. J. Inf. Manag. **36**(4), 557–569 (2016)

19. Durst, S., Edvardsson, I.R.: Knowledge management in SMEs: a literature review. J. Knowl. Manag. **16**(6), 879–903 (2012)

20. Harrison, R., Flood, D., Duce, D.: Usability of mobile applications: literature review and rationale for a new usability model. J. Interact. Sci. **1**(1), 1–16 (2013)

21. Shu-Sheng, L., Hatala, M., Huang, H.-M.: Investigating acceptance toward mobile learning to assist individual knowledge management: based on activity theory approach. Comput. Educ. **54**(2), 446–454 (2010)

22. Park, S.Y., Nam, M.-W., Seung-Bong, C.: University students' behavioral intention to use mobile learning: evaluating the technology acceptance model. Br. J. Edu. Technol. **43**(4), 592–605 (2012)

23. Cheon, J., Lee, S., Crooks, S.M., Song, J.: An investigation of mobile learning readiness in higher education based on the theory of planned behavior. Comput. Educ. **59**(3), 1054–1064 (2012). https://doi.org/10.1016/j.compedu.2012.04.015

24. Park, E., Baek, S., Ohm, J., Chang, H.J.: Determinants of player acceptance of mobile social network games: an application of extended technology acceptance model. Telematics Inform. **31**, 3–15 (2014)

25. Burney, S.A., Ali, S.A., Ejaz, A., Siddiqui, F.A.: Discovering the correlation between technology acceptance model and usability. Int. J. Comput. Sci. Netw. Secur. **17**(11), 53–61 (2017)

26. Praveena, K., Thomas, S.: Continuance intention to use Facebook: a study of perceived enjoyment and TAM. Int. J. Ind. Eng. Manag. Sci. **4**(1), 24–29 (2014). https://doi.org/10.9756/BIJIEMS.4794

27. Echeng, R., Usoro, A.: Enhancing the use of web 2.0 technologies in higher education: students' and lectures' views. J. Int. Technol. Inf. Manag. **25**(1), 89–106 (2016)

28. McKenna, B., Tuunanen, T., Gardner, L.: Consumers' adoption of information services. Inf. Manag. **50**(5), 248–257 (2013)

29. Chiu, C.M., Wang, E.T.G.: Understanding web-based learning continuance intention: the role of subjective task value. Inf. Manag. **45**(3), 194–201 (2008)

30. Venkatesh, V., Morris, M.G., Davis, G.B., Davis, F.D.: User acceptance of information technology: toward a unified view. MIS Q. **27**(3), 425–478 (2003)

31. Al Awadhi, S., Morris, A.: The use of the UTAUT model in the adoption of e-government services in Kuwait. In: Proceedings of the 41st Annual Hawaii International Conference on System Sciences, p. 219 (2008)

32. Nassuora, A.B.: Students acceptance of mobile learning for higher education in Saudi Arabia. Int. J. Learn. Manag. Syst. **1**, 1–9 (2013)

33. Hadie, S.N.H., Yusoff, M.S.B.: Assessing the validity of the cognitive load scale in a problem-based learning setting. J. Taibah Univ. Med. Sci. **11**(3), 194–202 (2016)

34. Wang, T., Jung, C.H., Kang, M.H., Chung, Y.S.: Exploring determinants of adoption intentions towards enterprise 2.0 applications: an empirical study. Behav. Inf. Technol. **33**(10), 1048–1064 (2014). https://doi.org/10.1080/0144929x.2013.781221

35. Anderson, J.C., Gerbing, D.W.: Structural equation modeling in practice: a review and recommended two-step approach. Psychol. Bull. **103**, 411–423 (1988)

36. McDonald, R.P., Ho, M.H.: Principles and practice in reporting structural equation analysis. Psychol. Methods **7**(1), 64–82 (2002)

37. Cronbach, L.J., Shavelson, R.J.: My current thoughts on coefficient alpha and successor procedures. Educ. Psychol. Measur. **64**(3), 391–418 (2004)

38. Sekaran, U., Bougie, R.: Research Methods for Business: A Skill Building Approach, 7th edn. Wiley, Hoboken (2016)

39. Cronbach, L.J.: Coefficient alpha and the internal structure of tests. Psychometrika **16**(3), 297–334 (1951). https://doi.org/10.1007/BF02310555

Health Informatics and Life-Long-Learning

Model-Based Diagnosis with FTTell: Assessing the Potential for Pediatric Failure to Thrive (FTT) During the Perinatal Stage

Natali Levi-Soskin[1](✉), Ron Shaoul[2,3], Hanan Kohen[1],
Ahmad Jbara[1,4], and Dov Dori[1,5]

[1] Faculty of Industrial Engineering and Management, Technion,
Israel Institute of Technology, Haifa, Israel
natali.levi@campus.technion.ac.il,
{hanank,dori}@technion.ac.il, ahmadjbara@gmail.com
[2] Ruth Children's Hospital, Rambam, Health Care Campus, Haifa, Israel
r_shaoul@rambam.health.gov.il
[3] Faculty of Medicine, Technion, Israel Institute of Technology, Haifa, Israel
[4] School of Computer and Cyber Sciences, Augusta University,
Augusta, GA, USA
[5] Systems Design and Management, Massachusetts Institute of Technology,
Cambridge, MA, USA

Abstract. Models have traditionally been mostly either prescriptive, expressing the function, structure and behavior of a system-to-be, or descriptive, specifying a system so it can be understood and analyzed. In this work, we offer a third kind —diagnostic models. We have built a model for assessing potential pediatric failure to thrive (FTT) during the perinatal stage. Although FTT is commonly found in young children and has been studied extensively, the exact etiology is often not clear. The ideal solution is for a pediatrician to input pertinent data and information in a single tool in order to obtain some assessment on the potential etiology. We present FTTell—an executable model-based medical knowledge aggregation and diagnosis tool, in which the qualitative considerations and quantitative parameters of the problem are modeled using a Methodical Approach to Executable Integrative Modeling (MAXIM)—an extended version of Object-Process Methodology (OPM) ISO 19450, focusing on the perinatal stage. The efficacy of the tool is demonstrated on three real-life cases, and the tool's diagnosis outcomes may be compared with and critiqued by a domain expert.

Keywords: Failure to thrive (FTT) potential · Executable models · Systems and software engineering · OPM ISO 19450 · Model-based diagnosis

1 Introduction

Medical knowledge in general and pediatric medical knowledge in particular have been increasing significantly over the past decades. Therefore, it is hard or maybe even impossible for a pediatrician to be updated even in her or his field of expertise. In an

© Springer Nature Switzerland AG 2019
S. Wrycza and J. Maślankowski (Eds.): SIGSAND/PLAIS 2019, LNBIP 359, pp. 37–47, 2019.
https://doi.org/10.1007/978-3-030-29608-7_4

attempt to provide a solution, some medical knowledge has been translated into computer interpretable formats as models or pseudo-code. Examples include GLIF [1], Arden [2], PROforma [3], EON [4], and GLARE [5]. The major problem with these frameworks is that they are not intuitive, and therefore medical doctors find them difficult to use. A 2016-published executable tool for representing medical knowledge and treatment protocols [6], which, to the best of our knowledge, is the state-of-the-art, translates medical data into Statechart models using the open-source tool Yakindu [7]. Since this tool is not executable and therefore does not provide for verification, an additional tool, Y2U [8], translates the Statecharts model from Yakindu to UPPAAL timed automata. In order to use this framework, medical doctors have to build the Statecharts model using Yakindu, then run Y2U to transform the model to UPPAAL timed automata, which can finally be executed, usually requiring help from a computer professional. Any change in the input data or the model structure, mandates updating the Statecharts model, re-running the Y2U tool, and executing the UPPAAL timed automata.

As the etiology of FTT is not well defined and has no consensus, models are subject to frequent changes. New factors might dynamically be added and existing ones might be changed or removed. Such modifications affect the model structure and will eventually invalidate the dynamic part due to lack of synchronization. The dynamic nature of FTT makes it difficult to develop a long-term write-once tool. A single tool that is based on a simple, coherent methodology, rather than a chain of disparate tools, will enable medical doctors to be actively involved in the tool development and its tuning as new factors and considerations emerge. Based on this motivation and our experience from previous works, including [9] and [10], we developed FTTell—a model-based improved, simple "one-stop-shop" medical diagnosis tool for assessing ("Telling") the potential for pediatric FTT during the perinatal stage. While different reasons may cause a child to deviate from the normal stature or weight for age and gender, it is not always the case that low weight or stature implies that a child fails to thrive [11, 12], as some of the reasons may be genetic- or nutrition-related. To diagnose FTT, the pediatrician should examine the child from many aspects, including parental (deprivation syndrome), prenatal growth, birth weight, and postnatal growth. Information about the parents, such as their heights, mother's nutrition status, and her emotional stress during the pregnancy, are also highly relevant. Our model represents succinctly and consistently the knowledge about the child at the perinatal stage—the period immediately before and after birth. It provides for collecting the required data, including the weight and length at different pregnancy stages, and getting an assessment of the child's FTT potential. Since diagnosis of FTT involves both qualitative and quantitative aspects, we have used MAXIM [10], an extension of OPM. OPM [13, 14], is an ISO 19450 [15] model-based systems and software engineering language and methodology. Using MAXIM, we can represent qualitative and quantitative data in a model and execute it.

The main contribution of this research is the prototype model-based FTT diagnostic tool, which automates and expands FTT assessment. The tool uses data from an often-ignored and not thoroughly explored period—the perinatal stage, which is fed into a single executable model. Once any member of the medical staff has inserted the required data into the model, that member can easily execute the model in a single step, watch the results, track and analyze issues, and let the pediatric expert use it as a decision-support tool with no need for a computer professional's help. The model can be easily updated and synchronized with new relevant data and knowledge that is likely to emerge as the research on FTT is evolving.

The structure of the rest of this paper is as follows. In Sect. 2, we present MAXIM, which includes OPM and its computational extension, as well as the OPCloud OPM modeling environment. In Sect. 3, we present the model of the perinatal stage for diagnosing FTT. We present both the main diagram, in which the pediatrician can insert the required data and watch the results after model execution. Also presented are the refined diagrams, in which intermediate calculations are made and can be watched for deeper investigation. In Sect. 4, we summarize this research and suggest future research directions.

2 Method and Tools

For developing FTTell we use MAXIM. MAXIM is based on OPM [13, 14] ISO 19450:2015 with extensions for computations. OPM, with its MAXIM extension, is a systems modeling approach [15] that represents the function, structure and behavior of any system using only two kinds of things (Fig. 1): objects—things that exist, and processes—things that transform objects.

Fig. 1. Example of an OPM object (left) and process (right)

Things can be physical (shaded) or informatical (not shaded). An informatical object can be valued, i.e., have a value, in which case it can also have units of measurement and an alias—a short, space-less name for use in formulae (see Fig. 2).

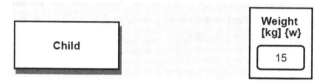

Fig. 2. An OPM physical object that represents a Child (left) and OPM informatical and computational object that represents a Weight of 15 kg and can be used in a formula shortly using its alias "w"

A process can be computational, in which case it accepts one or more object values as input parameters and performs a specified computation to produce a resulting object value. The difference between a physical process and an informatical and computational process is shown in Fig. 3.

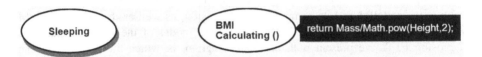

Fig. 3. The OPM physical process **Sleeping** (left) and the computational process **BMI Calculating** (right), which gets two valued objects, **Mass** and **Height** (not shown), and outputs a resulting value, the BMI object (not shown). The code of the computational process on the right appears in OPCloud while hovering over the process.

OPM things are connected by links, which graphically express relations. Any OPM model consists of two parts: (1) the OPD set: a set of Object Process Diagrams (OPDs) and, (2) the OPL spec: a collection of sentences in a subset of English (or any other natural language), called Object Process Language (OPL). Each OPD construct—things connected by links—is reflected as one or more OPL sentences. This bimodal representation caters to the dual channel assumption [16, 17]: the brain process information via both a visual and a verbal cognitive channels.

An OPM model can be presented at various levels of detail in different, interconnected views, each being an OPD. The top-level OPD is called System Diagram—SD, which usually consists of one systemic process and its operand – the object which that process transforms. Together, the process and the operand are the function of the system. Each OPD can be refined in one of several ways in order to expose deeper levels of detail. In this work, we use only process in-zooming to show subprocesses, of which the main process consists, and their temporal (sequential or parallel) execution order. MAXIM is developed and implemented as part of OPCloud [18], a collaborative cloud-based software environment for OPM-based modeling.

3   FTTell – Our OPM Model-Based FTT Diagnosis Tool

We start constructing our model by defining the main process, **Failure To Thrive (FTT) Diagnosing & Treating**, which is physical, as denoted in Fig. 4 by the shading of the ellipse representing this process.

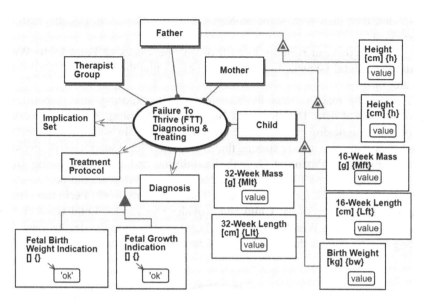

Fig. 4. SD of the FTTell system, showing the main process which is called **Failure To Thrive (FTT) Diagnosing & Treating**, the involved object set that serve as agents, and resulting objects

The **Failure To Thrive (FTT) Diagnosing & Treating** process involves the objects **Child, Mother, Father**, and **Therapist Group.** Each one of the is a physical object, connected to the main process by an agent link—a line with a black lollipop on its process end. OPM agents are humans involved in the process. The **Failure To Thrive (FTT) Diagnosing & Treating** process outputs three results: **Diagnosis, Treatment Protocol**, and **Implication Set.** Each result is represented by an object connected to the main process by a result link, as shown in Fig. 4.

The height of the child's parents can affect the FTT potential decision, so the **Mother** and **Father** have each a **Height** attribute. As Fig. 4 shows, **Height** is a computational object with cm units and the alias h. The mother's and father's **Height** attribute objects are respectively connected to the **Mother** and **Father** by an exhibition-characterization link, serving as input values. The object **Child** has five perinatal-related input attributes: **Mass** [g] and **Length** [cm] at **16-weeks** and **32-weeks** pregnancy, as well as **Birth Weight** [kg].

The final result of the model execution is the informatical objects **Fetal Birth Weight Indication** and **Fetal Growth Indication**, which are parts of the **Diagnosis** informatical object. This is expressed in Fig. 4 by aggregation-participation links—the lines with the black triangle in the middle. For the **Fetal Birth Weight Indication** object there are two possible result values: 'ok' and 'low'. For the **Fetal Growth Indication** object there are four possible values: 'ok', 'mother-dependent', 'mother- and child-dependent' and 'child dependent'. A result with value 'ok' means that there were no growth issues during the pregnancy. However, if the result is one of the other three options, then there were some problems, and an indication of possible reasons is then provided.

The small arrowhead pointing to each one of the values of **Fetal Birth Weight Indication** and **Fetal Growth Indication** symbolizes that these are the default values, which are 'ok'.

We refine the main process by zooming into it, exposing three subprocesses: **Diagnosing**, **Treatment Defining**, and **Implication Defining**. As in this work we focus on the **Diagnosing** process, we move on to Fig. 5, in which we refine **Diagnosing** by zooming into it and exposing three new, lower-level subprocesses: **Perinatal Growth Examining**, **Postnatal Growth Examining**, and **FTT Diagnosing Determining**. For diagnosing FTT, both perinatal and postnatal data should be considered, but here we focus on the former, leaving the latter for future work. **Perinatal Growth Examining** uses data from the **Child** and provides two results: **Fetal Growth Indication** and **Fetal Birth Weight Indication**. These objects have the default value 'ok', indicating that by default the growth and the birth weight of the fetus were normal.

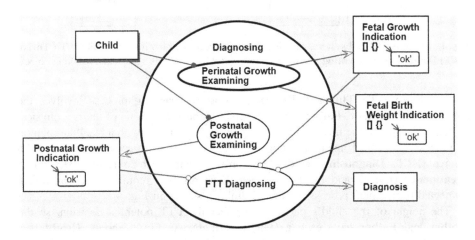

Fig. 5. SD1.1 - diagnosing in-zoomed

Finally, in Fig. 6, we zoom into the **Perinatal Growth Examining** process to determine the FTT potential. To this end, we calculate the ponderal index (PI) at 16 and 32 weeks, using the corresponding fetal **Mass** and **Length** at these time points while considering **Birth Weight** [11]. To perform these calculations, we wrote software code in OPCloud using the Typescript programming language.

The mathematical formula of PI is:

$$PI = \frac{mass(g)}{length(cm^3)} \times 100$$

The first subprocess, **First Trimester PI Calculating** (), gets as input two values: **16-week Mass** {Mft} and **16-week Length** {Lft}. The result is written into the output object **First Trimester PI** {PIft}. The Typescript code is:

```
return (Mft/Math.pow(Lft, 3))*100;
```

Last Trimester PI Calculating () has a similar structure, using as inputs **32-week Mass** {Mlt} and **32-week Length** {Llt}, so the code for calculating **Last Trimester PI** {PIlt} is:

```
return (Mlt/Math.pow(Llt, 3))*100;
```

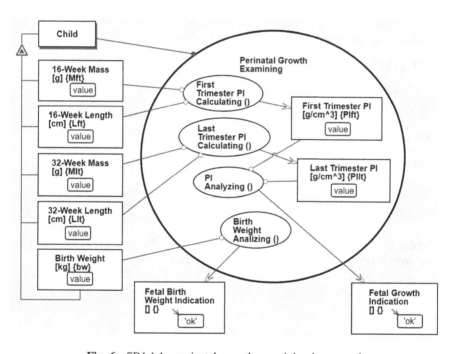

Fig. 6. SD1.1.1 - perinatal growth examining in-zoomed

To assess the FTT potential, **PI Analyzing** () gets as input PIft and PIlt, and the result can be one of the following: (1) 'ok', which means no FTT, (2) 'mother-dependent', which can result from causes such as the mother's stress or bad nutrition during pregnancy, (3) 'mother- and child-dependent', i.e., FTT is caused by both the mother and some problem with fetal development, and (4) 'child-dependent', implying a fetal development problem, such as lack of proteins. The program code of this process is:

```
let ft = true, lt = true;
let result = 'ok';
if (PIft<2.32 || PIft>2.85) {
    ft = false;
}
if (PIlt<2.32 || PIlt>2.85) {
    lt = false;
}
if (!ft) {
    result = 'mother-dependent';
    if (!lt) {
    result = 'mother- and child-dependent';
    }
} else if (!lt) {
    result = 'child-dependent';
}
return result;
```

Finally, the **Birth Weight Analyzing** () process uses the input **Birth Weight** {bw}, and the output is 'low' if the birth weight is less than 2.5 kg:

```
if (bw < 2.500) {
return 'low';
} else {
return 'ok';
}
```

Having developed and validated the FTTell model, we inserted into it the required data of each specific child, one at a time. The data is simulated, and was generated to test the efficacy of the FTTell system. Clicking on the execution button, we can follow tokens running visually through the different OPDs in a depth-first manner. Finally, the result values are updated in the model and can be exported to an Excel file.

Table 1 presents the results of particular data sets of three babies after executing the model. These are saved in an Excel file for documentation and can further serve for statistical analysis.

Table 1. Model execution results as saved in an Excel file

Fetal birth weight indication	Fetal growth indication	Birth weight	Last trimester PI	First trimester PI	32-week length	32-week mass	16-week length	16-week mass	
Ok	Ok	3.4	2.2	6.4	42.4	1702	11.6	100	Baby #1
Low	Ok	2.4	2.2	6.4	42.4	1702	11.6	100	Baby #2
Low	Mother- and child-dependent	2.4	2.3	2.9	41.3	1600	14	79.2	Baby #3

The first baby, Baby #1, was born with a weigh of 3.4 kg. It had a weight of 100 g and a length of 11.6 cm as a 16-weeks fetus, and a weight of 1702 g and a length of 42.4 cm as a 32-weeks fetus. This baby is defined as normal, with no FTT suspected. Baby #2 has the same pregnancy values but a low birth weight of 2.4 kg, so it is classified by the system as 'ok' in the **Fetal Growth Indication** parameter, but as 'low' in the **Fetal Birth Weight Indication** parameter. Therefore, it may have some FTT suspicion and should be under follow-up. However, there is a chance that this baby's weight will catch up with the normal one in the next growth interval. Baby #3 has low length and mass values during the different perinatal stages, and is classified by the system with **Fetal Growth Indication** value 'mother- and child-dependent'. This result is determined by calculating PI values and analyzing them. Bad PI values at the 16-week pregnancy time point are usually due to mother-related reasons, such as bad nutrition and stress. Bad PI values at the 32-week pregnancy time point are caused usually by child-related reasons, which can be genetic causes, malnutrition, or lack of proteins. In addition, the third baby has a low birth weight. For all these reasons, it has high chances to suffer from FTT and has to be checked by an expert.

4   Conclusions and Future Work

Conceptual models have been used mostly for descriptive or prescriptive purposes, serving for understanding and specifying phenomena and systems, respectively. In this research, we propose using a diagnostic model – the application of conceptual modeling for the purpose of medical diagnosis. Currently, high-quality diagnosis of FTT potential depends on the experience and expertise of the pediatrician. Hence, as a proof-of-concept to our diagnostic modeling approach, we have developed, implemented, and started to test FTTell – a model-based diagnosis system for FTT potential assessment. To this end, we used MAXIM—an extended version of OPM ISO 19450, augmented with computational capabilities and implemented as part of OPCloud. Using this cloud-based modeling environment has enabled us to transition back-and-forth between qualitative and quantitative modeling in a seamless and effortless fashion. The underlying FTTell model embeds the necessary procedures and computations required for an objective decision-making process that a pediatric expert would perform. The input needed for the computation is easy to insert, and the execution is done by a click of a button in a friendly user interface.

Since OPCloud is a cloud-based tool and can be accessed from anywhere, the software is "zero client", making it executable from anywhere and at any time. Future research can take several directions: (1) Extend FTTell to include the postnatal stage, add input reasons that would yield mother-related FTT indications, and model an individually adapted treatment protocol that accounts for each child's data and indications. (2) Modify the model-based diagnostic approach to additional medical conditions and diseases that similarly require a stepwise procedure and computations using data supplied by the medical expert. (3) Apply a similar approach to the diagnosis of failure causes of technological products and systems, and how to repair or treat them.

Acknowledgments. The research in this paper was partially funded by the Gordon Center for Systems Engineering at the Technion, Israel Institute for Technology.

References

1. Greenes, R.A., Tu, S., Boxwala, A.A., Peleg, M., Shortliffe, E.H.: Toward a shared representation of clinical trial protocols: application of the GLIF guideline modeling framework. In: Silva, J.S., et al. (eds.) Cancer Informatics, pp. 212–228. Springer, New York (2002). https://doi.org/10.1007/978-1-4613-0063-2_19
2. Pryor, T.A., Hripcsak, G.: The arden syntax for medical logic modules. Int. J. Clin. Monit. Comput. **10**(4), 215–224 (1993)
3. Fox, J., Johns, N., Rahmanzadeh, A.: Disseminating medical knowledge: the PRO forma approach. Artif. Intell. Med. **14**(1–2), 157–182 (1998)
4. Tu, S.W., Musen, M.A.: Modeling data and knowledge in the EON guideline architecture. Stud. Health Technol. Inform. **84**, 280–284 (2001)
5. Terenziani, P., Montani, S., Bottrighi, A., Torchio, M., Molino, G., Correndo, G.: The GLARE approach to clinical guidelines: main features. Stud. Health Technol. Inform. **101**, 162–166 (2004)
6. Guo, C., Ren, S., Jiang, Y., Wu, P.L., Sha, L., Berlin, R.B.: Transforming medical best practice guidelines to executable and verifiable statechart models. In: 2016 ACM/IEEE 7th International Conference on Cyber-Physical Systems, ICCPS 2016 (2016)
7. YAKINDU Statechart Tools. https://www.itemis.com/en/yakindu/state-machine/
8. Y2U (2009). http://www.cs.iit.edu/~code/software/Y2U/
9. Li, L., Levi-Soskin, N., Jbara, A., Karpe, M., Dori, D.: Model-based systems engineering for aircraft design with dynamic landing constraints using object-process methodology. IEEE Access **7**, 1 (2019)
10. Levi-Soskin, N., Marwedel, S., Jbara, A., Dori, D.: Towards Fusing Systems and Software Engineering : A Methodical Approach to Executable Integrative Modeling (Submitted for publication)
11. Schwartz, I.D.: Failure to thrive: an old nemesis in the new millennium. Pediatr. Rev. **21**(8), 257–264 (2007)

12. Mei, Z., Grummer-Strawn, L.M., Thompson, D., Dietz, W.H.: Shifts in percentiles of growth during early childhood: analysis of longitudinal data from the california child health and development study. Pediatrics **113**(6), e617–e627 (2004)
13. Dori, D.: Model-Based Systems Engineering with OPM and SysML. Springer, New York (2016). https://doi.org/10.1007/978-1-4939-3295-5
14. Dov, D.: Object-Process Methodology: A Holistic Systems Paradigm, 1st edn. Springer, Heidelberg (2002). https://doi.org/10.1007/978-3-642-56209-9
15. ISO/PAS 19450 Automation systems and integration – Object-Process Methodology (2015). https://www.iso.org/standard/62274.html
16. Mayer, R.E., Moreno, R.: Nine ways to reduce cognitive load in multimedia learning. Educ. Psychol. **38**(1), 43–52 (2003)
17. Mayer, R.E.: The promise of multimedia learning: using the same instructional design methods across different media. Learn. Instr. **13**(2), 125–139 (2003)
18. OPCloud. https://www.opcloud.tech/

Supporting Active and Healthy Ageing by ICT Solutions: Preliminary Lessons Learned from Polish, Swedish and Latvian Older Adults

Ewa Soja[1]([⊠]), Piotr Soja[2], Ella Kolkowska[3], and Marite Kirikova[4]

[1] Department of Demography, Cracow University of Economics,
Kraków, Poland
Ewa.Soja@uek.krakow.pl
[2] Department of Computer Science, Cracow University of Economics,
Kraków, Poland
Piotr.Soja@uek.krakow.pl
[3] Center for Empirical Research in Information Systems (CERIS),
Örebro University School of Business, Örebro, Sweden
Ella.Kolkowska@oru.se
[4] Department of Artificial Intelligence and Systems Engineering,
Institute of Applied Computer Systems, Riga Technical University, Riga, Latvia
Marite.Kirikova@cs.rtu.lv

Abstract. Since the growing amount of elderly people in the population is a challenge for most of the European countries, it would be favorable to develop models and processes for elderly care and healthcare based on the new digital solutions. However the social, economic and cultural environment differ between countries in Europe and it is important to acknowledge and understand the country-specific context when new digital solutions are implemented. The aim of this paper is to investigate older adults' needs and attitudes towards ICT solutions for independent living in three European countries: Sweden, Poland and Latvia. The study was conducted with the help of a questionnaire distributed to older adults in three regions in Sweden, Poland and Latvia. The results show that older adults in Sweden have greater requirements than respondents in Poland and Latvia regarding aspects important for satisfying and independent ageing. With respect to digital technologies supporting independent and healthy ageing, Polish respondents recognized that all such technologies should be developed; Latvians were more moderate in their opinions, while Swedish respondents were the most selective in their declarations.

Keywords: ICT · Active and healthy ageing · Poland · Latvia · Sweden

1 Introduction

Nowadays, population ageing, defined as an increase in the share of older people in the population, is a typical phenomenon of developed countries. According to demographic forecasts, in the case of European countries, the process of populations ageing will deepen in time [4]. Growing number of elderly in the population increases the

© Springer Nature Switzerland AG 2019
S. Wrycza and J. Maślankowski (Eds.): SIGSAND/PLAIS 2019, LNBIP 359, pp. 48–61, 2019.
https://doi.org/10.1007/978-3-030-29608-7_5

burden on health and care systems and families. To counteract the effects of an ageing population various strategies are suggested, among which the policy of active ageing appears to be the most crucial [26]. These strategies should enable and promote (1) longer working lives, (2) ensure that private family transfers are integrated into old-age security systems where possible, (3) promote well-being and (4) enable healthy and active living to reduce chronic illness and health care costs, and support active contributory life for as long as possible [9].

ICT is an extremely important element of the modern world, offering a wide range of potential benefits for organizations, individuals and the whole society. It can be a key tool in the development of the so-called silver economy, supporting the implementation of active and healthy ageing at the same time, transforming the challenges of ageing societies into opportunities for their development [10, 22]. Designing new, more holistic models for social care and healthcare that would take into account ageing in place and take advantage of new digital solutions is a one of prioritized areas in Europe [e.g. 16].

However, the use of the ICT-enabled opportunities does not look the same for all countries. This is due to different levels of digital inclusion of society, e.g. extent of digitization of businesses, digitization of public services, deployment of broadband infrastructure or skills needed to use the possibilities offered by the digital society [2, 13]. Countries may also differ with respect to the social and healthcare system, which is manifested in the level of implementation of the policy of active and healthy ageing (e.g. possibilities to access to health services, independent living, financial security and health status, and digital inclusion of the elderly) [22, 28].

For instance Patomella et al. [14] investigated everyday technology use among older adults in Sweden and Portugal. The authors argue that studying technology use in general is important for understanding how older adults engage in everyday occupations and ageing in place. They also found that there were significant differences between the studied countries regarding the kind and the number of everyday technologies considered as important, which is stemming mostly from different socio-economic and technology levels. With this respect, previous research suggests that the use of ICT in transition countries, i.e. countries who are transitioning or recently transitioned from centrally planned economy to a free market system, is characterized by different considerations than in the most developed countries. As a result, the use of existing models and theories, most of which have been developed in the context of the most developed countries of the world, has a limited application in the case of transition economies [18]. We argue that to be able to take advantage of other countries' experiences and attain user acceptance that is necessary to achieve the benefits of modern ICT solutions, it is important to acknowledge and understand country-specific differences especially between western European countries and eastern European countries [23].

The aim of this paper is to investigate older adults' needs and attitudes towards ICT solutions for independent living in three European countries: Sweden, Poland and Latvian. These three countries appear more diverse with respect to the level of digital development [20]. However, Poland and Latvia appear similar to each other as regards the level of the implementation of strategy for active and healthy ageing. They also reveal the considerations of transition economies [10, 22]. This study seeks to answer the following research questions: *(1) What factors are important for the older adults in Sweden, Poland and Latvia to have an independent and satisfying life as people age? (2) What kind of digital technology needs to be developed to support independent and healthy ageing according to older adults in Sweden, Poland and in Latvia?*

The rest of the paper is structured as follows. In the next section we describe the background for this study. After that we present our research method followed by the presentation of the results. The paper ends with a discussion and conclusions.

2 Background

Europe has a rapidly ageing population because of an increased longevity combined with falling fertility. According to UN projections [24], the share of people aged 65 years and more will increase from 2015 year to 2045 by about 9%. At the same time, the potential labor resources in group age 20–64 years will fall by 8%. The expected demographic changes will also affect the populations of Sweden, Poland and Latvia, with more severe consequences for transition economies (Poland and Latvia) (Table 1). The needs of ageing population will be challenging for society because of a strong increase in people no longer working, often in need of long-term health and social care, combined with an imbalance between active and inactive people, and a lack of (formal and informal) caregivers [4].

Table 1. Percentage of total population by age group

Year:	2015	2045	2015–2045	2015	2045	2015–2045	2015	2045	2015–2045
Age:	20–64			50–64			65+		
Europe	61,5%	53,4%	−8,1%	20,5%	19,6%	−0,9%	17,6%	26,9%	9,3%
Latvia	61,2%	54,3%	−6,9%	20,6%	21,6%	1,0%	19,3%	26,6%	7,3%
Poland	64,2%	55,4%	−8,8%	20,9%	23,6%	2,7%	15,6%	28,5%	12,9%
Sweden	57,9%	53,8%	−4,1%	17,9%	18,5%	0,6%	19,6%	24,1%	4,5%

Source: Own elaboration based on [24]

One of the strategies that aim at maintaining the well-being and social security of ageing societies is the concept of active ageing. It is understood as the process of optimizing opportunities for maintaining activity, independence and health to improve the quality of life over the years [3, 26]. However, European countries differ in the degree of implementation of active and healthy ageing strategies. The Active Ageing Index (AAI) is a measure constructed to evaluate current activities and to set targets and monitor progress towards this policy in future [27]. AAI consists of components representing four domains of assessment: employment, social activity and independent living of older adults, and the ability of the environment to implement active ageing. For example, a domain independent living relates to access to health services or financial security. With this respect, the Swedish system is built on state responsibility model with strong emphasis on redistribution, social inclusion and universality of public services. In Poland and Latvia, only some of the care needs are satisfied by the government, while other services are rendered by families and private service organizations [e.g. 5, 10, 17].

Previous research based of the AAI and cluster analysis, showed, that Poland and Latvia and most of the countries undergoing economic transformation formed a separate group, characterized by a relatively higher evaluation of employment and the lowest assessments of other domains. A separate group was formed by the Scandinavian countries, so also Sweden, together with Ireland and the United Kingdom, with the highest marks in all areas [22].

Differences in the level of implementation of active and healthy ageing strategies in the countries under examination, especially in the area related to independent ageing, can affect the perception of the needs related to independent living as people age and perception of ICT solutions that support such life. This problem is important because the majority of older adults would like to live independently in their own places of residence, as long as it is possible [19]. This way of living by the elderly (so-called ageing in place) is also recommended by decision makers and institutions dealing with social and health care due to financial (avoiding expensive institutional care) and psychosocial benefits for people who want to maintain their autonomy and independence by getting support in his own home [7, 16].

Generally, ICT is seen as a powerful means to support such kind of living of elderly as well as a possibility to empower people of every age to better manage their health and quality of life and, as a consequence, to maintain cost efficiency and have high quality health and social care. ICT solutions can, for instance, remind a user about taking medicine, help to structure the day for a person with cognitive decline, send medical data to a responsible physician who can immediately react on undesirable changes in the elderly health status. By aiding communication with relatives, healthcare and homecare, ICT can increase the sense of safety and security as well as reduce loneliness and social exclusion.

However, it appears that possibilities of using ICT for active and healthy ageing depend largely on the level of development of digital economy and society [12, 13]. As mentioned above, current activities toward strategy of active and healthy ageing are captured by the AAI. Digital Economy and Society Index (DESI), in turn, measures the level of development of digital economy and society [1]. This indicator is a weighted average of indexes describing the following components (domains): Connectivity (infrastructure and its quality), Human Capital (skills), Use of Internet, Integration of Digital Technology, and Digital Public Services. Rankings of European countries by the level of DESI and AAI were largely consistent; it was confirmed by the value of Spearmen rank correlation coefficient (0.76) for these indexes [22].

In order to evaluate the differences in the level of digitalization of economy and society of European countries, including Sweden, Latvia and Poland, a cluster analysis has been performed. Two agglomeration methods have been used: the hierarchical Ward's method and non-hierarchical k-means method [6]. In consequence, three groups of countries similar with respect to the assessment of individual domains were identified (Table 2). Table 2 presents country groups with distances from the cluster centre for each country.

Table 2. Clusters of countries obtained with the use of the k-means method for DESI

Cluster 1		Cluster 2		Cluster 3	
AT	0,010	BE	0,015	BG	0,009
CZ	0,013	DK	0,014	HR	0,017
EE	0,020	FI	0,015	CY	0,009
FR	0,009	LU	0,020	EL	0,009
DE	0,019	NL	0,009	IT	0,009
HU	0,017	**SE**	0,011	**PL**	0,014
IE	0,018	UK	0,018	RO	0,019
LV	0,017				
LT	0,018				
MT	0,013				
PT	0,019				
SK	0,017				
SI	0,009				
ES	0,010				

The analysis of the mean values of standardized domain-specific DESI indexes calculated for each cluster, displayed in Fig. 1, allowed us to identify the nature of the country groups. The third group is characterized by the lowest values of all domains of DESI. Poland belongs to this group. The first group, comprising Latvia, is characterized by somewhat greater levels of all domains as compared to the third group. The second group, in turn, is comprised of countries which achieved the highest values of all domain-specific indexes and Sweden belongs to this group. Particularly great differences between the groups, and thus the investigated counties, are visible for domains Connectivity and Human Capital, which measure the deployment of broadband infrastructure and its quality, and the skills needed to use the possibilities offered by the digital society. This might have an influence on individual perceptions of ICT solutions for supporting independent and active life.

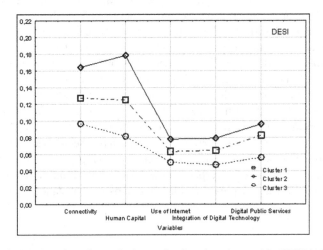

Fig. 1. Mean values for each cluster for five domain-specific DESI indexes

Summing up, previous research indicates that there may be many factors affecting the acceptance and use of ICT solutions to support active and healthy life. To use the experience of other countries and create solutions that increase user acceptance, it is important to recognize and understand individual and country-specific considerations. When examining them, one should take into account both the specific personal context concerning the elderly (e.g. needs related to independent living or attitudes towards using ICT) as well as technological/digital factors and socio-economic determinants [e.g. 11, 15].

3   Research Method

In our study, we focused on the investigation of the opinions of the older adults concerning the needs related to independent living and the attitudes towards using ICT. For this purpose we used the data from the preliminary survey which was conducted with the help of a questionnaire distributed to older adults aged 50 to 89 years in three regions in three countries: Sweden (Örebro County), Poland (Krakow and its surroundings), and Latvia (Riga and its surroundings). Questions were asked in two categories. The first category included questions related to the needs which are considered by the respondents to be important for an independent and satisfying life as people age. The factors that the respondents could select within the first category were:

1. ability to choose where they will live (e.g. independently at home, at home with family, nursing home, at home with help coming); this factor was named "type of residence",
2. ability to choose what they will eat ("kind of food"),
3. ability to choose when they will eat ("time of meals"),
4. ability to be outside when and as much as they want ("time in outdoors"),
5. ability to participate in cultural activities (e.g. theater, cinema, concerts – "cultural activity"),
6. ability to perform physical activity ("physical activity"),
7. ability to decide what kind of help they will receive (e.g. personal care, cleaning, shopping – "kind of aid"),
8. ability to choose the time of assistance ("time of aid"),
9. ability to choose the assisting person ("assisting person").

The second category included questions about the types of ICT solutions that according to respondents should be developed to support independent and healthy ageing. Examples of digital technologies that the respondents could select within the second category were:

1. robots assisting independent eating (this device was named as "eating"),
2. technologies facilitating communication (e.g. with family, health care, care – "communication"),

3. memory-supporting technology ("memory"),
4. health monitoring technologies (e.g. remote transmission of blood pressure measurement, sugar level – "health monitoring"),
5. technology that help with personal hygiene ("hygiene"),
6. cleaning robots ("cleaning"),
7. monitoring and alarming technologies (e.g. fall detection – "alarming").

In both categories the respondents were also asked to indicate their suggestions regarding what is important for a satisfying life and what technological solutions should be developed.

All items were measured on a three-point Likert-type scale: 3 – very important, 2 – important, and 1 – not important. On the basis of the values extracted from the respondent answers, synthetic scores for variables were calculated. The scores were weighted average values, where the percentages of answers to individual questions were adopted as weights.

The Swedish sample consisted of 409 people (median age = 68), the Polish sample counted 470 people (median age = 67), and the Latvian sample consisted of 315 respondents (median age = 68). The oldest age group in the Swedish sample and the middle groups in the Polish and Latvian samples were overrepresented. Therefore, in the final analysis, we used appropriate weights for these samples. The adopted weights took into account the proportions in the age and gender structure of the analyzed populations. In doing so, for each country, the 10 years-long age groups within the analyzed populations aged 50–89 were taken into consideration.

4 Results

In the case of the first question, the results show that for the majority Polish, Latvian and Swedish older adults all of the indicated factors were important for having a meaningful everyday life as people age (Fig. 2). However, the perception of the importance of the different factors varies from country to country. This is also indicated by the synthetic evaluations of the importance of individual factors illustrated in Fig. 3. In general, older adults in Sweden considered the factors more important than older people in Poland and in Latvia. At the same time, Latvian respondents included the greatest percentage of answers indicating the factors as unimportant.

In Sweden, six for all nine factors received synthetic scores close to 3 points ("type of residence", "kind of aid", "time of aid", assisting person", "time in outdoors", "kind of food"), which indicates that these were very important for the vast majority of respondents, while in Poland only two factors with averages 2.7 ("kind of food") and 2.6 ("time in outdoors") were perceived as very important by the vast majority of older adults. In the case of Latvia, only one factor with an average 2.6 ("type of residence") was assessed as very important for the vast majority of respondents. Ability to choose where who will live in the future ("type of residence") was the only common, the most important factor in all countries. It should be noted, however, that no one identified this factor as not important in Sweden, but in Poland this option was indicated by 2% of respondents and even 9% of respondents in Latvia.

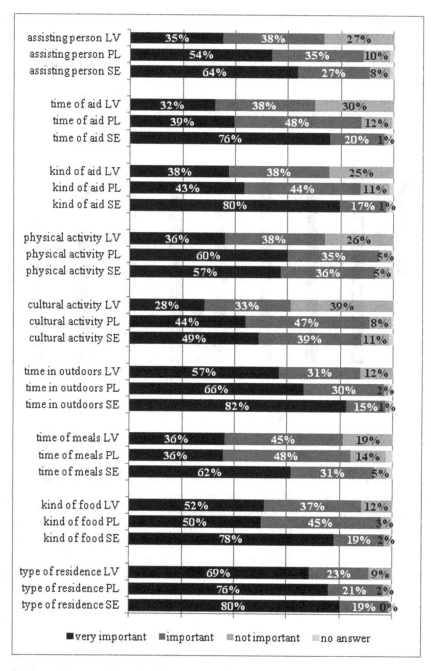

Fig. 2. Answers to questions about the importance of factors for independent and satisfying life as people age in Sweden (SE), Poland (PL) and Latvia (LV)

Participation in cultural and recreational activities obtained the lowest synthetic scores in all countries, which means that this factor was less important for the majority of respondents. In the case of Latvia, almost 40% of respondents considered it as not important. It should be added that at least 25% of Latvian older adults indicated also as irrelevant factors such as "time of aid", "kind of aid", "assisting person" and "physical activity". They were also slightly less appreciated by Poles, except "physical activity", with was very important for 60% of respondents (this was even more than in Sweden).

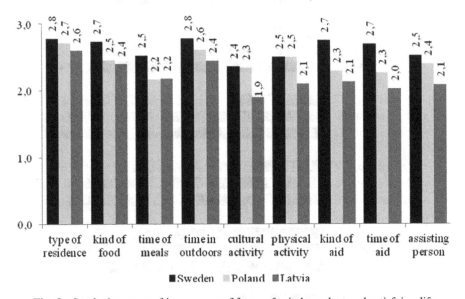

Fig. 3. Synthetic scores of importance of factors for independent and satisfying life

Regarding older adults' attitudes to development of technology supporting independent ageing, we found both some similarities and differences between the studied countries (Figs. 4 and 5). Poles, Latvians and Swedes were together stronger interested in developing solutions facilitating communication, memory-supporting technology, health monitoring technologies, and monitoring and alarming technologies. All synthetic scores for these technologies received values of at least 2, except for the evaluation of "health monitoring" for Sweden, which, however, was very close to 2. In the case of other solutions, the significant differences were visible. The vast majority of Swedish respondents did not perceive the importance of developing technologies facilitating eating and cleaning. Nevertheless, Swedes to a moderate extent supported development of technologies facilitating personal hygiene. The majority of Latvians did not support the necessity of developing robots assisting independent eating, however, they supported development of technology that help with personal hygiene and support cleaning. Older adults in Poland, in turn, indicated the need for development of technologies facilitating personal hygiene, cleaning, and eating. Only 30% of Poles expressed a clear negative attitude toward robots facilitating eating and

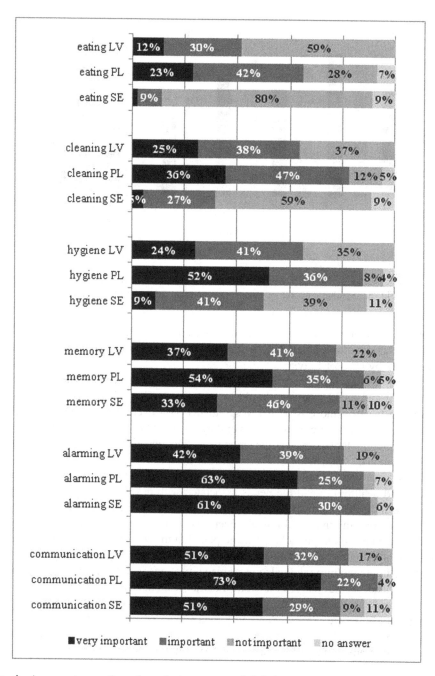

Fig. 4. Answers to questions about the importance of digital technologies according to Swedish (SE), Polish (PL) and Latvian (LV) older adults

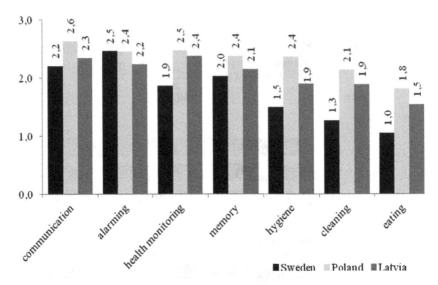

Fig. 5. Synthetic scores of importance of factors for digital technologies

considered development of these technologies as not important. It was definitely different in other countries, where such negative opinions were expressed by even 80% of Swedes and by 60% of Latvians.

Generally, Poles have recognized that all kinds of digital technologies supporting independent and healthy ageing should be developed. The opinions of Latvian were more moderate than those of Polish respondents. However, the recommendations of Swedish respondents were more selective: they supported development of the majority of the proposed solutions and, at the same time, they negated the need for developing certain solutions.

Taking into considerations individual suggestions of respondents regarding independent and healthy life and the needs associated with developing other technologies than those indicated, it should be noted that the number of opinions was not great. However, among the indicated issues, several positions were repeatedly declared and they conceivably should be included while planning the solutions for the future. Poles, Latvians and Swedes together drew mainly attention to the need of developing solutions to facilitate mobility; they also recognized meetings with family and friends as an important need. Additionally, Polish and Latvian respondents pointed to the need for better medical care. Older adults in Poland indicated also the possibility of participating in religious life, whereas respondents in Latvia suggested the need for Internet access and older Swedes paid attention to computer games that could be used for entertainment, social interaction and for improving concentration and memory.

5   Discussion and Conclusion

The results of our research suggest the existence of a certain pattern associated with the level of implementation of active and healthy ageing and the level of digital development of economy and society. It seems that older adults in Poland and Latvia have lower requirements than Swedes regarding the factors needed for a satisfying and independent ageing. It appears that these differences might depend on individual experience in elderly care and possibility of realization of needs associated with independent life. Both Poland and Latvia belonged to the group of countries where activities for social participation and independent living of older adults and capacity for active ageing were very limited, which is indicated by the values of AAI domains. Sweden, in turn, belonged to the leaders in this field. In particular, it appears that different models for elderly care, which in Poland and Latvia were primarily based on family care, could lower requirements or anxiety about the quality of aid. However, it should be emphasized that in all countries older adults considered the ability to choose the type of residence as a very important factor for independent and successful ageing.

In the case of ICT solutions for independent and healthy ageing, older adults in Poland are the most interested in their development. On the one hand, this may be due to the generally lower level of digitalization of economy and society than in Latvia and Sweden, and hence the need for its development. On the other hand, Poles are aware that due to the existing care system they will need to rely on themselves or on their families when they get older. Therefore, they hope that modern technologies will help them to be able to cope with everyday life at home when they get older. Such an explanation appears coherent with the results achieved for Latvia with respect to solutions useful for health problems (health monitoring) or for handicapped people (robots supporting eating and cleaning), which were similar to results obtained for Poland and were significantly different from the findings achieved for Sweden. The current elderly and health care systems in Poland and Latvia were similar; they did not provide sufficient help for the elderly with health problems, which was also reflected in individually reported needs associated with the improvement of medical services.

In the case of Sweden, greater experience and knowledge of the possibilities of modern technologies to support independent and healthy life, resulting from a better implemented strategy of active ageing and higher development of digitalization, allows older adults to more knowingly (selectivity) present their current needs. Because the health condition of Swedes is relatively better than the health condition of Poles and Latvians [20], and in the case of disability they can count on state aid, therefore they are significantly interested in developing alarming technology (most from all countries) or communication technology, but they do not support the necessity of technology development facilitating food or cleaning.

The results of our research illustrate some avenues for future investigations. In particular, in further research it is worth considering whether the requirements and opinions of respondents change with age and gender. In the case of Poland, gender-related differences were confirmed in Soja's research [21]; however, they were related to the Polish care system. It is also worth taking into account the division into gender, as previous studies indicate that women are more often involved in providing help to the elderly [8]. Also, prior research suggests that there may be differences in attitudes towards ICT between women and men [25].

The current study contributes to research by providing an increased understanding of how needs and attitudes towards ICT solutions supporting independent living may differ in different socioeconomic settings. In consequence, the achieved results might help in development of sustainable solutions that are more relevant to local contexts and are accepted by senior users. This suggests that strategies and ICT solutions for active and healthy ageing cannot be just transferred between countries in Europe without reflection and adaptation of the solutions to the specific country context.

Acknowledgments. This research has been financed in part by The Swedish Institute, Sweden, and the funds granted to the Faculty of Management, Cracow University of Economics, Poland, within the subsidy for maintaining research potential.

References

1. European Commission: DESI 2017 Digital Economy and Society Index Methodological note (2017). https://ec.europa.eu/digital-single-market/en/desi
2. European Commission: The 2018 Ageing Report. Underlying Assumptions and Projection Methodologies. European Economy Institutional Paper 065 (2017)
3. European Commission: Growing the European Silver Economy (2015). http://ec.europa.eu/research/innovation-union/pdf/active-healthy-ageing/silvereco.pdf
4. European Commission: The 2015 Ageing Report. Economic and budgetary projections for the 28 EU Member States (2013–2060). European Economy 3 (2015)
5. European Commission: Access to healthcare and long-term care: Equal for women and men? Final synthesis report. Publications Office of the European Union, Luxembourg (2010)
6. Everitt, B.S., Landau, S., Leese, M.: Cluster Analysis. Edward Arnold, London (2001)
7. Golinowska, S.: The Present and Future of Long-Term Care in Ageing Poland. The World Bank (2015). https://das.mpips.gov.pl/source/opiekasenioralna/Long%20term%20care%20in%20ageing%20Poland_ENG_FINAL.pdf
8. Haberkern, K., Schmid, T., Szydlik, M.: Gender differences in intergenerational care in European welfare states. Ageing Soc. **35**(2), 298–320 (2015)
9. Harper, S.: Economic and social implications of aging societies. Science **346**(6209), 587–591 (2014)
10. Klimczuk, A.: Comparative analysis of national and regional models of the silver economy in the European Union. Int. J. Ageing Later Life **10**(2), 31–59 (2016)
11. Kolkowska, E., Avatare Nöu, A., Sjölinder, M., Scandurra, I.: Socio-technical challenges in implementation of monitoring technologies in elderly care. In: Zhou, J., Salvendy, G. (eds.) ITAP 2016. LNCS, vol. 9755, pp. 45–56. Springer, Cham (2016). https://doi.org/10.1007/978-3-319-39949-2_5
12. Kolkowska, E., Soja, E., Soja, P.: ICT for active and healthy ageing: comparing value-based objectives between polish and swedish young adults. In: Proceedings of the International Conference on ICT Management for Global Competitiveness and Economic Growth in Emerging Economies (ICTM 2018), pp. 39–49. University of Wrocław, Wrocław (2018)

13. Kolkowska, E., Soja, E., Soja, P.: Implementation of ICT for active and healthy ageing: comparing value-based objectives between polish and swedish seniors. In: Wrycza, S., Maślankowski, J. (eds.) SIGSAND/PLAIS 2018. LNBIP, vol. 333, pp. 161–173. Springer, Cham (2018). https://doi.org/10.1007/978-3-030-00060-8_12

14. Patomella, A.-H., Kottorp, A., Ferreira, M., Rosenberg, L., Uppgard, B., Nygård, L.: Everyday technology use among older adults in Sweden and Portugal. Scand. J. Occup. Ther. **25**(6), 436–445 (2017)

15. Peek, S.T.M., et al.: Older adults' reasons for using technology while aging in place. Gerontology **62**(2), 226–237 (2016)

16. Rigby, M., Koch, S., Keeling, D., Hill, P., Alonso, A., Maeckelberghe, E.: Developing a New Understanding of Enabling Health and Wellbeing in Europe: Harmonising Health and Social Care Delivery and Informatics Support to Ensure Holistic Care. European Science Foundation, Strasbourg, France (2013)

17. Rosochacka-Gmitrzak, M., Racław, M.: Opieka nad zależnymi osobami starszymi w rodzinie: Ryzyko i ambiwalencja. Studia Socjologiczne **2**(217), 23–47 (2015)

18. Roztocki, N., Weistroffer, H.R.: Information and communication technology in transition economies: an assessment of research trends. Inf. Technol. Dev. **21**(3), 330–364 (2015)

19. Sixsmith, J., et al.: Healthy ageing and home: the perspectives of very old people in five European countries. Soc. Sci. Med. **106**, 1–9 (2014)

20. Soja, E.: Supporting healthcare of the elderly through ICT: socio-demographic conditions and digital inclusion. In: Malina, A., Węgrzyn, R. (eds.) Knowledge, Economy, Society: Challenges and Development of Modern Finance and Information Technology in Changing Market Conditions, pp. 279–289. Foundation of the Cracow University of Economics, Kraków (2016)

21. Soja, E.: Information and communication technology in active and healthy ageing: exploring risks from multi-generation perspective. Inf. Syst. Manag. **34**(4), 320–332 (2017)

22. Soja, E.: Supporting active ageing: challenges and opportunities for information and communication technology. Zarządzanie i Finanse J. Manag. Finance **15**(1/2017), 109–125 (2017)

23. Soja, P., Cunha, P.R.: ICT in transition economies: narrowing the research gap to developed countries. Inf. Technol. Dev. **21**(3), 323–329 (2015)

24. United Nations: Department of Economic and Social Affairs, Population Division World Population Prospects: The 2017 Revision (2017)

25. Wagner, N., Hassanein, K., Head, M.: Computer use by older adults: a multi-disciplinary review. Comput. Hum. Behav. **26**(5), 870–882 (2010)

26. Walker, A., Maltby, T.: Active ageing: a strategic policy solution to demographic ageing in the European Union. Int. J. Soc. Welfare **21**(1), 117–130 (2012)

27. Zaidi, A., Gasior, K., Zolyomi, E., Schmidt, A., Rodrigues, R., Marin, B.: Measuring active and healthy ageing in Europe. J. Eur. Soc. Policy **27**(2), 138–157 (2017)

28. Zaidi, A., Stanton, D.: Active Ageing Index 2014: Analytical Report. UNECE, European Commission (2015)

3D Authoring Tool for Blended Learning

Andrew Zaliwski[1(✉)] and Karishma Kelsey[2]

[1] Whitireia Polytechnic, Auckland CBD, New Zealand
Andrew.Zaliwski@Whitireia.ac.nz
[2] Karishma Design, Auckland, New Zealand
karishmadesign@gmail.com

Abstract. Over the last years, a growing interest in blended learning, that can be defined as the mixing of online courses with face-to-face courses taking advantage of both worlds [7, 17, 33], has been on the increase.

This paper proposes a computerized tool for collaborative *authoring of revitalized reusable teaching modules (so-called learning objects – LO) for blended learning*. The tool will orchestrate the timing of various classroom activities (e.g. multimedia presentations, team activities, case studies, etc.) and can assist with the way how a learning management system (e.g. Moodle) interact with students. The tool also addresses the need for collaboration when several teachers work on the development of the same course offered at more than one branch of the college. While trying to fill up the gap between objects storage and retrieval standards and the object's usage in the class context under given learning theory based on constructivism and connectionism, the paper also presents visual metaphors for the described authoring tool.

The tool is assumed to save the teacher's time and energy to make teaching more effective.

Keywords: Blended learning · 3D learning objects authoring ·
Pedagogical context · Connectionism · Constructivism

1 Introduction

Teachers prepare students for a changing world where rapid changes in technologies create an impression of uncontrolled change. Where some jobs vanished due to AI, and some new, previously unknown jobs arise. New information systems supporting new business models enabled by new technologies require a new approach. The old model of profit-based business and economy becomes obsolete when confronted with new challenges like social enterprise, emerging "sharing" economy, circular economy, co-building value with customers (and competitors), and pairing business sustainability along with environmental sustainability, etc.

For example [5]: "The amount of new technical information is doubling every two years. For students starting a 4-year technical college degree, this means that half of what they learn in their first year of study will be outdated by their third year of study". Hopefully, new teaching paradigms are not based on remembering information, but rather on using them.

© Springer Nature Switzerland AG 2019
S. Wrycza and J. Maślankowski (Eds.): SIGSAND/PLAIS 2019, LNBIP 359, pp. 62–73, 2019.
https://doi.org/10.1007/978-3-030-29608-7_6

According to Richard Riley, former US Secretary of Education [27]: "We are currently preparing students for jobs that don't yet exist, using technologies that haven't yet been invented, in order to solve problems, we don't even know are problems yet."

The preparation of professionals further working in this environment is also challenging. Teaching models [8, 32] are no longer based on transfer knowledge ex-cathedra but are flexible where the teacher may provide autonomy for learners in material selection, however, limited to the sandbox of safe learning space where is no one is drifting into the wrong direction.

The process of course stream preparation is usually messy, time-consuming, and needs hoarding of a number of potentially usable variants of learning materials. Business and IT courses (like e.g. System Analysis and Design, or business courses supporting Information Systems programs like "Organizational Change", or "Project Management" for example) should be deeply rooted into the contemporary business needs, trends, and requirements) more and more often use the newest video clips, case studies and other examples from the real life and business practice, and references to the lastly published business papers related to the topic presented by the teacher. This kind of courses needs to be systematically adapted to changing social, political, technological, and economic conditions (reflecting changes in the business environment) to illustrate the course concepts by the last events.

Additionally, courses may contain reusable pieces shared with other courses (e.g. in different studies program offerings). Natural borders between teaching domains become porous, some topics are repeated on several different courses (e.g. SWOT analysis, research methods, (e.g. on strategic management, international marketing, marketing communication, e-Business, etc.).

We need fast creation and combining of different streams of teaching materials into the cohesive stream which can be delivered into the classroom along with the synchronized activities building social and innovative skills among multicultural students, building environmental awareness along with standard business knowledge – teaching co-operation and design win-win situations both for people, business, and environment.

Usually, tertiary institutions have several branches offering the same course. This requires collaborative work on the course material. This requires employing the concepts of learning object and cloud-based learning object repository maybe with versioning of the subsequent solutions.

The purpose of the course authoring tool proposed in this paper is the production of a logical sequence of "containers" with course materials, which will be delivered according to the current course schedule. The word "logical" in this context means that delivery of the course materials will be controlled by a number of constraints (e.g. new materials will be built upon the previous one, not using terms not defined earlier).

Note that each "container" being a course delivery unit may contain an arbitrary number of learning objects, not making any earlier assumptions on the learning objects standards. This should allow for further cooperation with other tools and systems based on learning objects through the creation of proprietary interfaces.

The proposed approach should allow teachers to smoothly to face incoming challenges faced by educators [20]:

- the current teaching process should be rather focused on developing various forms of participation and negotiation among teachers and students, rather than giving direction and instruction by the teacher;
- creating a more sophisticated, integrated learning mix;
- navigating and seeing the knowledge network is at least as important as knowing facts;
- using richer assessments and evaluations;
- dealing with the emergence of the new pedagogies;

Section 2 of this paper summarize two basic building blocks used to create our solution: *blended learning* and *learning objects*. Section 3 adds additional building blocks in the form of teaching theories like *constructivism* and *connectivism*.

2 Literature Review

2.1 Blended Learning

According to the Queensland University of Technology (2011): "Blended learning is a practical framework that can be used to encapsulate a range of effective approaches to learning and teaching. It encourages the use of contemporary technologies to enhance learning, and the development of flexible approaches to course design to enhance student engagement." The second concept which is utilized in this paper is the concept of the learning object, which is defined as "a blend of learning concepts and the computer science's object-orientation that defines an object as self-describing. It includes all the information about itself and can be located anytime. An object can be used in various settings [34].

Students who participated in blended learning courses appreciate this way of teaching due to their added value as flexibility, better support, better interaction and communication [12–14, 16]. It also has been proven [3, 28, 39], that transition from face-to-face learning to instruction based on reusable learning objects (LO) is effective and profitable for all teaching institution stakeholders, having economic and social benefits to society [4], improves learning outcomes, increases student satisfaction and student's engagement [15, 17, 41, 44].

The success of blended learning depends on the availability of high-quality content (frequently represented as reusable learning objects) on one side and on the pedagogical context (based on learning theory and learning process definitions and activities) on the other side.

2.2 Learning Objects

The learning objects (LO) brings a promise of reducing the costs of education by reuse education materials. There exist several definitions of learning objects e.g. IEEE definition [25] or [45–47].

The current model of learning objects is not sufficient to create complete units of study deliverable through a learning management system. Friesen [15] after examination of the e-learning standards of several institutions responsible for establishing standards like e.g. IEEE LTSC (Institute of Electrical and Electronics Engineers, Inc. Learning Technology Standards Committee), and the ISO/IEC have found that the e-learning standards are created primarily to solve technical rather than pedagogy issues. Similarly, Blandin [2]: From the one side, to maintain learning objects reusability, the LO should be as neutral as possible, from the other side, fully neutral learning objects are difficult for pedagogical use. This problem may be solved by creating pedagogically meaningful objects by combining a set of more or less neutral objects. However, the "Connecting LO to the instructional theory" remains a research problem [45–47].

3   The Authoring Process

The authoring process will follow the scenario:

- Pick-up everything what seems to be usable into the number of containers related to main course topics. In other words, search the Internet for usable information (find several alternatives for the same topics) or just pick-up everything that seems to be usable.
- Each container now may contain one or more learning objects (LO). Each LO should contain a complete program for the self-standing lesson (several of these lessons may be delivered during one class unit).
- Create a constrained network of containers showing dependencies among them. Some materials cannot be presented before the others. This may be several parallel paths between the containers.
- Define a set of alternative paths for material presentation leading from the beginning to the end of the network.
- Pick-up one delivery path through the network (among the others possible) which fit your situation and schedule it over the course timetable.
- Each learning object in the container is self-standing and it is delivered at the same time but each part of it by the different delivery channels. In other words, the LO contains current material of the lesson with presentation (supported by handouts and pre-existing Moodle or Blackboard materials, mobile delivery, interactive games, etc.) which should be delivered, with links to appropriate related video materials, and along with the in-class activities to perform during the class time. Orchestrated delivery of all materials to perform planned lesson in a synchronized way.

The whole above process is defined upon two teaching theories: connectivism and constructivism. The details are presented in the next section.

4   Theoretical Background

The proposed system is built-up upon two learning theories:

- The connectivism theory used for gathering and combining the course building blocks into a network of knowledge (taking into account different variants and alternative versions of some collected materials).

- The constructivism theory is used for graphical interactive extraction of one most sensible path among many alternatives – a stream defining the sequence of course activities delivery.

To create meaningful pedagogical material the teacher or designer uses by-products from various sources of information. The information is coming from various unstructured or structured mostly internet sources. This cannot be mistaken with knowledge. Ability to find required or usable information doesn't mean the practical, profitable, and effective use of it. The learning designer should have the ability to search and navigate among accessible information and next use the collected information to design a final stream of teaching materials which will be delivered to target audience using principles of constructivism.

To realize this, we analyze the everyday operations and behavior of a teacher when preparing a course, describing this initial process of information gathering in the notion of connectivism learning theory [9–11, 37, 42, 43] where:

- "Learning is understood as a process of connecting specialized nodes or information sources".
- Distinguishing between important and unimportant information is significant.
- "Ability to see connections between fields, ideas, and concepts is a core skill."
- "Learning may reside in non-human appliances" (e.g. artificial intelligence).
- "Capacity to know more is more critical than what is currently known"
- Nurturing and maintaining connections is needed to facilitate continual learning.
- Core skills are the ability to see connections between fields, ideas, and concepts.
- "The recognition when new information alters the landscape of yesterday is critical".
- "Decision-making is itself a learning process. Choosing what to learn and the meaning of incoming information is seen through the lens of a shifting reality. While there is a right answer now, it may be wrong tomorrow due to alterations in the information climate affecting the decision."

The business or IT problems specifics naturally dictate the use of (social) constructivism-based methods for teaching. Constructivism approach to learning supports the following teaching goals [24]:

- "Provide experience with the process of knowledge construction"
- "Provide experience in and appreciation for multiple perspectives"
- "Embed learning in real-life context" (for example the case methods).
- "Embed learning in social experience" (for example cultural sensitivity, storytelling [31]).
- "Support usage of multiple modes of representation"

The larger list of goals was presented by Murphy [38] and it was further extended by Koohang [34, 36]. Using constructivist theory to e-learning (and blended learning) is supported by the researchers [18, 40, 48, 49]. From a practical point of view the constructivist-based teaching may be characterized by three factors [6]:

- **"Active participation of the student in the learning process.** Knowledge acquisition requires the execution of programmed practical activities based on collaboration and cooperation among students where students' motivation decide about better participation."

- **"Interaction with other students."** Collaboration and cooperative activities develop social skills.
- **"Personalized learning environment.** A high affinity for learning content increases the student's motivation. That is, the learner is more motivated the better adapted is the content to his/her needs."

The pedagogically driven stream delivered to the student should also be structured, what means presented in the correct order from easier to more complicated topics, team assignment, case studies, task, and selected examples should stimulate learning. The creation of this stream is a task for learning designers.

The connectivism approach seems to be ideal to create a logically connected network from mostly unstructured input material. The connectivism learning theory is seen by some authors as a further development of constructivism [1, 26] by adding more focus on networks and connections [29].

The network may be employed to be a living representation of knowledge and navigated [19] by the learning designer to create the final version of a stream delivered to students. Constructivism learning theory by focusing on knowledge construction based on learner's previous experience is effective for e-learning [18, 22, 23, 35].

To summarize, the proposed tool described in the next chapter is a bridge between connectivism world (at the top general level – *what to teach*? In other words, "hoard whatever you think is usable to build-up course stream) and constructivism world (at the bottom detail level – *how to teach*? Organize what you have into logical stream delivered by different channels to the students).

5 The Network Editor

The first step of authoring is collecting (hoarding) the materials usable for teaching from the internet (Fig. 1A) and finally other sources to create a simple learning object (LO). The funnel (Fig. 1B) symbolizes the selection of usable course chunks from all available content. (There exists a solution for extracting learning objects which eventually may be considered here e.g. [30]). A network of related LO is created considering constraints based on prerequisites for the presentation of different parts of the material and eventually other constraints deciding about the order of LO. As a result of selection and applying constraints we have the networked structure (Figs. 1C and 2) of all usable course material. This is a number of alternate paths through the network. Any path from the start to the end point of the network is a valid course schedule, however with different alternative materials and with different level of difficulty.

The 3D view (Figs. 1D and 3) allows selecting alternative paths e.g. according to the difficulty of a given LO in the network. For example, more difficult LO can be placed higher on the 3D landscape. The connection between objects in 3D space represents various options for creating a final course schedule. To build up the schedule there is necessary to traverse a path through selected items on the network.

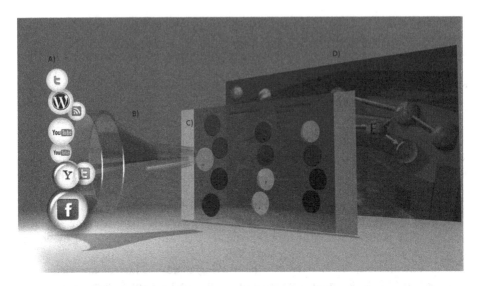

Fig. 1. The overall process of initial information gathering.

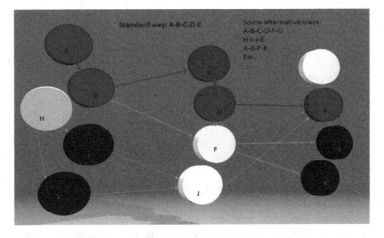

Fig. 2. A network of dependencies between course LO. The course material to be logical may be presented only on that time order (from left to right).

Course material is represented as a network of alternative teaching tracks (connecting LO in order of presentation) placed on different heights of a landscape representing the level of difficulty (Fig. 3). The result after selection of a path of course materials destined for course presentation in on Fig. 4. The previously selected stream of LO is packed into containers.

Each container is a course unit to be presented during one schedule unit (e.g. day or week). Each container contains one LO which was taken from the path determined in the previous step (Fig. 3) plus eventually any additional usable items (e.g. intentionally selected alternative LO from the alternative path).

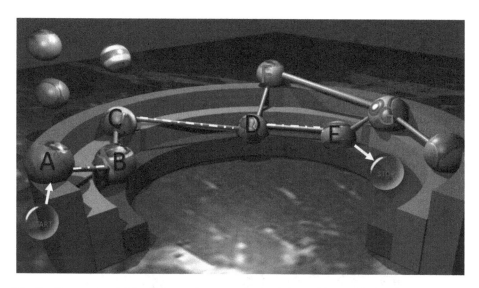

Fig. 3. Course material is represented as a network of alternative teaching tracks (connecting LO in order of presentation) placed on different heights of a landscape representing the level of difficulty (Source: Author [48]).

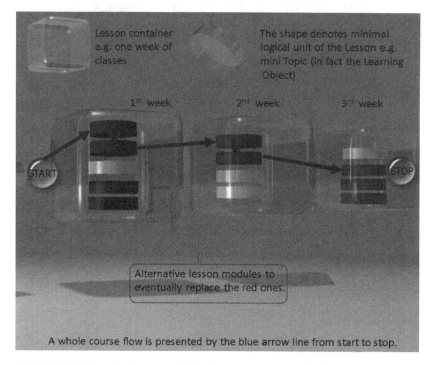

Fig. 4. The final shape of a course material selected into different containers (one container per course unit – in that case a week).

Each container is a compound construction (Fig. 5) which later can be broken into smaller pieces from which each of them can be delivered to the students in different ways (using various delivery channels e.g. Moodle, an in-class presentation, video, etc.). The items from the learning object are synchronized to be delivered at the same time. In other words, the items belonging to the same learning object, when the time comes to present those objects are delivered in different ways. For example, MS PowerPoint presentation from the current object A (Fig. 5) is delivered by the teacher (in-class presentation on Fig. 5), but at the same time on Moodle students have access to all related handouts coming from the same container for the current LO (Moodle channel on Fig. 5). The content of each learning object is delivered through the different channels in real time to the presentation of the specific corresponding LO (Fig. 6).

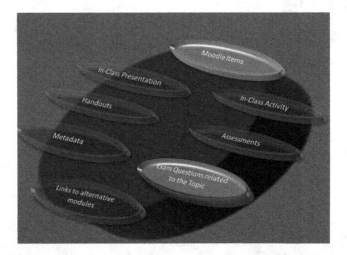

Fig. 5. The internal working structure of the container.

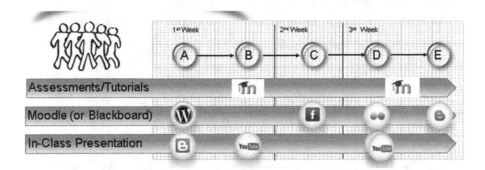

Fig. 6. The synchronized content delivery from the LO which is provided for presentation. On the picture is presented a timeline of the course containing a number of LO to present each week.

6 Further Research

The proposed tools may be recognized as a type of learning object (LO) production line, (the term pointed by Labib [21]) that covers the whole process of creating a course (or modifying of existing ones) in the form of an LO stream, where the LO is reusable course modules, set up in a co-operative manner.

Currently, the tool exists only as a proof of concept. It will be realized using the Blender 3D Game Engine with Python. The next stage will be finding the best usage of the tool. Followed by storing the prepared learning objects on a cloud repository to allow co-operation among the teachers teaching the same courses but at geographically different places.

Additionally, each learning object is itself a separate basket like Dropbox. Where different items from the internet may be just dropped if are usable for this part of the course. Another feature desired from each learning object is the ability for versioning the content. If the content was edited only the last version will be visible inside the container, however, several previous versions of the same material may be accessible at special request.

References

1. Bell, F.: Connectivism: its place in theory-informed research and innovation in technology-enabled learning. Int. Rev. Res. Open Distrib. Learn. **12**(3), 98–118 (2011)
2. Blandin, B.: Are e-learning standards neutral. In: International Conference on Computer Aided Learning in Engineering Education (2004)
3. Chan, D.: A comparison of traditional and blended learning in introductory principles of accounting course. Am. J. Bus. Educ. **4**(9), 1–10 (2011). https://www.academia.edu/6148679/A_Comparison_Of_Traditional_And_Blended_Learning_In_Introductory_Principles_of_Accounting_Course
4. Cohen, E., Nycz, M.: Learning objects and e-learning: an informing science perspective. Interdisc. J. E-Learning Learn. Objects **2**(1), 23–34 (2006). http://ijklo.org/Volume2/v2p023-034Cohen32.pdf
5. Corrigan, P.T.: Preparing students for what we can't prepare them for. Teaching & learning in higher ed (2013)
6. de-la-Fuente-Valentín, L., Pardo, A., Kloos, C.D.: Generic service integration in adaptive learning experiences using IMS learning design. Comput. Educ. **57**(1), 1160–1170 (2011)
7. Du, C.: A comparison of traditional and blended learning in introductory principles of accounting course. Am. J. Bus. Educ. **4**(9), 1–10 (2011)
8. Doue, W., Manning, D.K.: John Dewey and the art of teaching: toward reflective and imaginative practice. Educ. Found. **20**(3–4), 105–109 (2006)
9. Downes, S.: An Introduction to Connective Knowledge (2007). http://www.downes.ca/post/33034. In: Hug, T. (ed.) Media, Knowledge & Education-Exploring new Spaces, Relations and Dynamics in Digital Media Ecologies. Proceedings of the International Conference held on June 2007
10. Downes, S.: Learning Networks and Connective Knowledge (2006). http://it.coe.uga.edu/itforum/paper92/paper92.html
11. Downes, S.: What connectivism is (2007). http://halfanhour.blogspot.com/2007/02/what-connectivism-is.html

12. Fabry, D.L.: Using student online course evaluations to inform pedagogy. J. Res. Innov. Teach. **5**(1), 45–52 (2012)

13. Fearon, C., Starr, S., McLaughlin, H.: Value of blended learning in university and the workplace: some experiences of university students. Ind. Commer. Training **43**(7), 446–450 (2011). https://doi.org/10.1108/00197851111171872

14. Fearon, C., Starr, S., McLaughlin, H.: Blended learning in higher education (HE): conceptualising key strategic issues within a business school. Dev. Learn. Organ.: Int. J. **26** (2), 19–22 (2012). https://doi.org/10.1108/14777281211201196

15. Friesen, N.: Interoperability and learning objects: an overview of e-learning standardization. Interdisc. J. E-Learning Learn. Objects **1**(1), 23–31 (2005)

16. Garrison, D.R., Vaughan, N.D.: Blended Learning in Higher Education: Framework, Principles, and Guidelines. Wiley, Hoboken (2008)

17. Graham, C.R.: Blended learning systems. In: The Handbook of Blended Learning, pp. 3–21 (2006)

18. Harman, K., Koohang, A.: Discussion board: a learning object. Interdisc. J. E-Learning Learn. Objects **1**(1), 67–77 (2005). http://ijello.org/Volume1/v1p067-077Harman.pdf

19. Heylighen, F.: Structuring knowledge in a network of concepts. In: Workbook of the 1st Principia Cybernetica Workshop. Principia Cybernetica, Brussels (1991)

20. Hannon, V., Patton, A., Temperley, J.: Developing an innovation ecosystem for education. Cisco White Paper, December 2011

21. Labib, A.E., et al.: Enforcing reuse and customization in the development of learning objects: a product line approach. In: Proceedings of the 30th Annual ACM Symposium on Applied Computing. ACM (2015)

22. Hung, D.: Design principles for web-based learning: Implications from Vygotskian thought. Educ. Technol. **41**(3), 33–41 (2001)

23. Hung, D., Nichani, M.: Constructivism and e-learning: balancing between the individual and social levels of cognition. Educ. Technol. **41**(2), 40–44 (2001). https://repository.nie.edu.sg/bitstream/10497/14135/1/ERA-AME-AMIC-2000-144_a.pdf

24. Honebein, P.C.: Seven goals for the design of constructivist learning environments. In: Constructivist Learning Environments: Case Studies in Instructional Design, pp. 11–24 (1996)

25. IEEE Learning Technology Standards Committee (LTSC). Draft Standard for Learning Object Metadata Version 6.1 (2001). http://ltsc.ieee.org/wg12/

26. Goldie, J.G.S.: Connectivism: a knowledge learning theory for the digital age? Med. Teach. **38**(10), 1064–1069 (2016)

27. Gunderson, S., Roberts, J., Scanland, K.: The Jobs Revolution: Changing How America Works. Copywriters Incorporated (2004)

28. De Salas, K., Ellis, L.: The development and implementation of learning objects in a higher education setting. Interdisc. J. E-Learning Learn. Objects **2**(1), 1–22 (2006)

29. Del Moral, M.E., Cernea, A., Villalustre, L.: Connectivist learning objects and learning styles. Interdisc. J. E-Learning Learn. Objects **9**(1), 105–124 (2013)

30. Kawase, R., et al.: Openscout: harvesting business and management learning objects from the web of data. In: Proceedings of the 22nd International Conference on World Wide Web. ACM (2013)

31. Kelsey, K., Zaliwski, A.: Let's tell a story together. Interdisc. J. E-Learning Learn. Objects **13** (2017)

32. Kerr, B.: Which radical discontinuity. Recuperado el 30 (2007)

33. Khechine, H., et al.: UTAUT model for blended learning: the role of gender and age in the intention to use webinars. Interdisc. J. E-Learning Learn. Objects **10**(1), 33–52 (2014)

34. Koohang, A.: Creating learning objects in collaborative e-learning settings. Issues Inf. Syst. **4**(2), 584–590 (2004)
35. Koohang, A., Harman, K.: Open source: a metaphor for e-learning. Inform. Sci. **8**, 75–86 (2005)
36. Koohang, A., et al.: E-learning and constructivism: from theory to application. Interdisc. J. E-Learning Learn. Objects **5**(1), 91–109 (2009)
37. Kop, R., Hill, A.: Connectivism: learning theory of the future or vestige of the past? Int. Rev. Res. Open Distrib. Learn. **9**(3), 1–13 (2008)
38. Murphy, E.: Constructivism: From Philosophy to Practice (1997)
39. Matheos, K.: Innovative practices research project: COHERE report on blended learning. Ottawa, Canada: Human Resources and Skills Development Canada (2011). http://cohere.ca/wp-content/uploads/2011/11/REPORT-ON-BLENDED-LEARNING-FINAL1.pdf
40. Oliver, M., Trigwell, K.: Can 'blended learning' be redeemed? E-learning Digit. Media **2**(1), 17–26 (2005)
41. Sharpe, R., et al.: The undergraduate experience of blended e-learning: a review of UK literature and practice. High. Educ. Acad. 1–103 (2006)
42. Siemens, G.: Connectivism: A learning theory for the digital age (2004). http://www.itdl.org/Journal/Jan_05/article01.htm
43. Siemens, G.: Learning and knowing in networks: changing roles for educators and designers. ITFORUM Discuss. **27**, 1–26 (2008)
44. Vaughan, N.: Perspectives on blended learning in higher education. Int. J. E-learning **6**(1), 81–94 (2007)
45. Wiley, D.: Learning objects need instructional design theory. In: ASTD e-Learning Handbook, pp. 115–126 (2002)
46. Wiley, D.: Learning Objects need Instructional design (2000)
47. Wiley, D.A.: Connecting learning objects to instructional design theory: a definition, a metaphor, and a taxonomy. Instr. Use Learn. Objects **2830**(435), 1–35 (2000)
48. Zaliwski, A.J.: Collaborative authoring of Learning Objects for Blended Learning. eResearch Australasia 2010 (poster)
49. Zaliwski, A., Kelsey, K.: Building interaction with multicultural students - a fusion of multiple ancient and modern teaching technologies. In: The Third European Conference on Technology in the Classroom, IAFOR, Brighton, UK, 1–6 June 2015 (2015)

IT Security

DevSecOps Metrics

Luís Prates[1(✉)], João Faustino[1(✉)], Miguel Silva[1],
and Rúben Pereira[2(✉)]

[1] Instituto Universitário de Lisboa (ISCTE-IUL), Lisbon, Portugal
{lfbps, joao_faustino,
miguel_angelo_silva}@icste-iul.pt
[2] ISTAR-IUL, Instituto Universitário de Lisboa (ISCTE-IUL), Lisbon, Portugal
ruben.filipe.pereira@iscte-iul.pt

Abstract. DevSecOps is an emerging paradigm that breaks the Security Team Silo into the DevOps Methodology and adds security practices to the Software Development Cycle (SDL). Security practices in SDL are important to avoid data breaches, guarantee compliance with the law and is an obligation to protect customers data. This study aims to identify metrics teams can use to measure the effectiveness of DevSecOps methodology implementation inside organizations. To that end, we performed a Multivocal Literature Review (MLR), where we reviewed a selection of grey literature. Several metrics purposed by professionals to monitor DevSecOps were identified and listed.

Keywords: DevOps · DevSecOps · DevSecOps metrics · SecDevOps ·
Multivocal Literature Review

1 Introduction

Nowadays there is a trending methodology within Information Technology (IT) called DevOps that from a high-level perspective is defined has the merging of the Development team and Operations team into one. This methodology has proven productivity gains and DevOps professionals feel their work has more impact and it's recognized by all the organization [1]. DevOps increases both deployment frequency and the pace by which companies can serve their customers without compromising the quality of deliveries [2]. DevOps has indeed influenced software development but faster development cycles and increase of deployments that DevOps promises in conjunction with new engineering practices and tools may compromise security and this is discussed on research related with security aspects of DevOps [3] other research focus on security on CI/CD pipeline [4] from these researches the term DevSecOps and other aliases were coined [2]. DevSecOps is defined as the integration of security practices into DevOps [5]. This term is still recent but already is consider has topic having its own merit [2].

This research aims to study the scientific developments on DevSecOps and elicit a set of metrics grounded on professional and academics viewpoints, so organizations can monitor DevSecOps. Metrics are important to improve the rigor of measurement in both Software Engineering and Information systems fields and proposing such measures opens a debate for better understanding of the topic under discussion [6].

S. Wrycza and J. Maślankowski (Eds.): SIGSAND/PLAIS 2019, LNBIP 359, pp. 77–90, 2019.
https://doi.org/10.1007/978-3-030-29608-7_7

Since DevSecOps is a very recent topic the research methodology selected for this study is a MLR. MLR is a kind of Systematic Literature Review (SLR) [7] and is useful when trying to close the gap between academic research and professional practice [8].

The rest of this document is organized as such. Section 2 gives theoretical background on DevOps and DevSecOps, Sect. 3 describes the research methodology, Sect. 4 describes the literature review plan, Sect. 5 summarizes the information extracted from the analyzed publications, and discusses the results and limitations of the study, and Sect. 6 reports the findings and Sect. 7 concludes the paper.

2 Theoretical Background Review

2.1 DevOps

DevOps literature shows that defining the term has been hard. DevOps most typical description is Development plus Operations, but this description is not enough to explain DevOps [9]. Roche provides a good summary on the different viewpoints of what is DevOps. For some it is a specific job that requires development and IT operational skills for others DevOps is more than that [10]. Those who think that the term is more than a specific job defend the existence of four perspectives: collaboration, automation, sharing and measurement [11, 12]. DevOps is not only culture aspects it is also a set of engineering practices influenced by cultural aspects and supported by technological enablers [9]. DevOps capabilities are Continuous planning, Continuous integration and testing, Continuous release and deployment, Continuous infrastructure monitoring and optimization, Collaborative and continuous development, Continuous user behavior monitoring and feedback [9, 13].

DevOps is a complete new organizational mindset that replaces siloed units with cross-functional teams. DevOps achieves this by taking advantage of automated development, deployment, and infrastructure and enables teams to continuous work and deliver operational features [14].

2.2 DevSecOps

The same way that we can say DevOps is Development and Operations merged together we can say that DevSecOps is Development, Security and Operations merged together. DevSecOps is defined in literature as the integration of security processes and practices into DevOps environments and seen as a necessary expansion to DevOps [5].

The terms "DevSecOps", "SecDevOps", "SecOps", "RuggedOps", "Security in Continuous Delivery", and "Security in Continuous Deployment" are all aliases to DevSecOps [3]. In current literature is already possible to find a set of practices for DevSecOps [5]. Continuous Testing, Security as Code, Threat modelling, Risk analysis, Monitoring and logging and Red Team security drills. Continuous Testing is the practice of having automatic security controls throughout the software development lifecycle, continuously detecting for defects in code changes with the possibility of automatic rollback if necessary [5, 13]. Security as Code is the practice of having security policies like network configurations codified integrated with software development lifecycle [5]. Monitoring and logging practices is observing various quality parameters associated with the implemented controls and measure their effectiveness [5, 13]. Threat Modeling is the activity attacking your system on paper and using this information to identify, describe, and categorize threats to your system [3, 5]. Risk Analysis is the activity of creating security design specifications from the first planning and before every iteration [3, 5]. Red Team security drills is the practice of creating a proactive team that performs a malicious attack on deployed software with the intent of finding and exploiting vulnerabilities, finding security flaws and helping the organization find solutions [5, 15].

The two main benefits of DevSecOps are having fast and scalable security controls by Automating Security and having security controls since the beginning of the development process by Shifting Security to Left, this means bringing security experts involved from the beginning to plan and integrate security controls [5] but also to share knowledge with other team elements making them more security aware.

3 Research Methodology

This study follows a MLR methodology. A MLR is a form of a SLR which includes grey literature in addition to the published (formal) literature [7].

MLR in Software Engineering (SE) is not usual [7] and there are no guidelines to perform a MLR, since MLR is a form of SLR the review is planned as SLR but including "grey literature".

SLR is a type of literature review that is used to identify, evaluate and interpreting all available research relevant to a specific question [16]. Kitchenham's procedures for performing systematic reviews will be adopted by the authors. Figure 1 details how this research steps maps to the three phases proposed by Kitchenham [16].

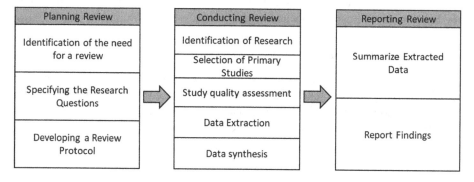

Fig. 1. MLR steps

Planning Review – this phase consists in three steps. First step is identifying the need and motivation for the review, second step is specifying the research questions that are going to be addressed and answered by the review. Final step designing a review protocol with the constraints that are going to be applied in the review. This phase is presented in Sect. 4.

Conducting Review – this phase consists in applying the designed review protocol. This phase is presented in Sect. 5.

Reporting Review – final phase of the review is summarizing the extracted data from the selected literature and report findings. This phase is presented in Sect. 6.

4   Planning the Review

This section details the first phase of the SLR. Motivation for this work is presented, followed by the Research Question this study intent to address and answer. Finally, Review Protocol is proposed.

4.1   Motivation

This research aims to study the scientific developments on DevSecOps and elicit a set of metrics grounded on professional and academics viewpoints, so organizations can monitor DevSecOps. Metrics are important to improve the rigor of measurement in both Software Engineering and Information systems fields and proposing such measures opens a debate for better understanding of the topic under discussion [6]. One of the principles found in DevOps and DevSecOps is measuring. DevSecOps encourages development of metrics that track threats and vulnerabilities throughout the software development lifecycle. Applying automatic security controls to the software development process provides development teams with metrics capable of tracking threats and vulnerabilities, allowing the organization with insights on the quality of software being developed [5].

Therefore, this work aims to obtain information about which metrics associated with DevSecOps are already identified by academics and professionals and the value they bring to development teams and organizations.

4.2   Research Questions

Based on what was described before it was established the importance of having metrics has way to better understand a topic under discussion for that reason the research aims to answer the following Research Question (RQ).

RQ: Which are the most relevant DevSecOps metrics.

4.3   Review Protocol

The first stage of the review protocol is literature search, a search string must be defined and applied in the chosen data sources with the intent of retrieving the highest possible number of studies related with the proposed research questions.

The search string is a set of keywords related to DevSecOps. Search terms used in this research are presented in Table 1.

Table 1. Search terms

Term	Keywords
DevSecOps or SecDevOps	Definition, Challenges, Metrics, Measuring, Adoption

The chosen academic data sources for the this MLR are three well-known academic databases.

- IEEEXplore (www.ieeexplore.ieee.org/Xplore/)
- ACM Digital Library (www.portal.acm.org/dl.cfm)
- SpringerLink (www.springerlink.com/)
- Google Scholar (https://scholar.google.com/)

For searching grey literature Google Search (www.google.com) was chosen.

Inclusion and exclusion criteria is applied to literature from both data sources. Criteria is presented in Table 2.

Table 2. Inclusion and exclusion criteria

Inclusion criteria	Exclusion criteria
Written in English	Not written in English
Publication date after 2013, inclusive	Publication date before 2013
Scientific papers in conferences or Journals, Blogs	Inaccessible literature
Explicit discusses DevSecOps	Duplicated
Limit results to first 3 pages of Google Search	Vendor tool advertisement Unidentified author No publication date

After applying the inclusion and exclusion criteria, remaining documents are read with the intent of obtaining the final selection of studies and at this point it's possible to conduct the review. The review protocol is represented in Fig. 2.

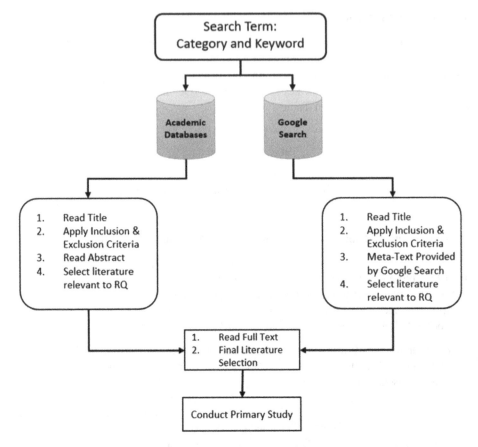

Fig. 2. Review protocol adapted from [5]

5   Conducting the Review

This section corresponds to second phase of the MLR and consists of applying the previously defined review protocol.

5.1   Selection of Studies

First step was to run the search string composed by the search terms defined on Table 1. After running the search terms on the selected data sources 558 articles were obtained. Distribution of articles by category is illustrated on Fig. 3 and by database illustrated on Fig. 4. The searches on the data sources only considered articles published after 2013.

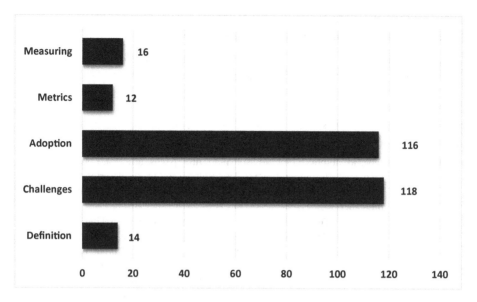

Fig. 3. Distribution of articles by search term

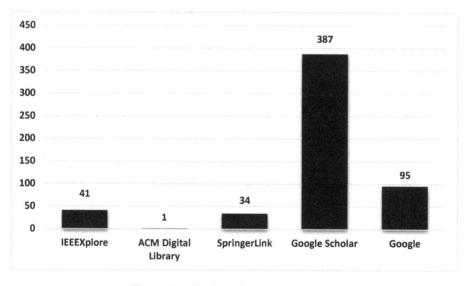

Fig. 4. Distribution of articles by database

Next step of the review protocol is applying the inclusion and exclusion criteria.

5.1.1 Academic Databases

First step is ensuring that there is not duplicated articles. Removing the duplicates consists on a two-step approach.

1. Remove Duplicates from articles retrieve from same database.
2. Remove Duplicates between the four academic databases.

Studies information exported from each data source were on different formats. Table 3 shows the export format from each academic data source.

Table 3. Academic databases export format.

Data source	Format
ACM	type, id, author, editor, advisor, note, title, pages, article_no, num_pages, keywords, doi, journal, issue_date, volume, issue_no, description, month, year, issn, booktitle, acronym, edition, isbn, conf_loc, publisher, publisher_loc
IEEE	Document Title, Authors, Author Affiliations, Publication Title, Date Added To Xplore, Publication_Year, Volume, Issue, Start Page, End Page, Abstract, ISSN, ISBNs, DOI, Funding Information, PDF Link, Author Keywords, IEEE Terms, INSPEC Controlled Terms, INSPEC Non-Controlled Terms, Mesh_Terms, Article Citation Count, Reference Count, Copyright Year, License, Online Date, Issue Date, Meeting Date, Publisher, Document Identifier
SpringerLink	Item Title, Publication Title, Book Series Title, Journal Volume, Journal Issue, Item DOI, Authors, Publication Year, URL, Content Type
Google Scholar	Title, Publication, Authors, Year

To ensure that the removal of duplicated studies is accurate, a database schema was created on PostgreSQL and a Table with the following attributes Title, Publication, Authors, Year were included since this are sufficient to identify a duplicated study. Insertion scripts that converted from the original format to the new database format were created for each data source, except for Google Scholar that already respected the desired format. After removing duplicated articles and applying the remaining items on the inclusion and exclusion criteria a total of 40 studies from academic databases were flagged as relevant to the research question. Table 4 details number of academic articles remaining after each phase.

Table 4. Academic articles remaining after each phase.

Phase	Number of articles
Duplicated	62
Read title	51
Inclusion & exclusion criteria	49
Read abstract	40
Full-text read and final selection	2

5.1.2   Grey Literature

The approach to filtering the grey literature is like the one used on the academic databases. First step is removing the duplicated, this was achieved by filtering duplicated URL's on Excel. After removing the duplicated articles, inclusion and exclusion criteria is applied a total of 56 were flagged as relevant to research question. Table 5 details number of grey literature articles remaining after each phase.

Table 5. Grey literature articles remaining after each phase.

Phase	Number of articles
Duplicated	234
Read title	92
Inclusion & exclusion criteria	65
Meta text provided by Google	56
Full-text read and final selection	11

5.1.3   Final Selection of Studies

From the pool of literature flagged as possible relevant to the research question, all texts were read to further decide the document's relevance, and a total of 13 were obtained as relevant to our study.

5.2   Data Extraction Analysis

Based on the obtained artefacts from this MLR there is little literature related with DevSecOps and in particularly on literature related in how organizations can measure the efficiency of DevSecOps implementations.

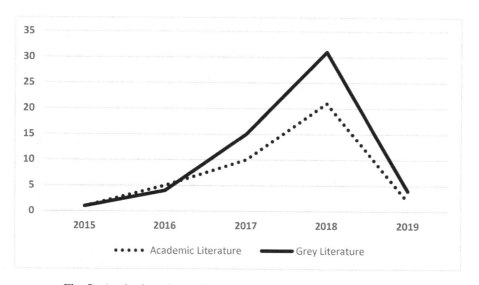

Fig. 5. Academic and grey literature articles flagged as relevant by year

Even so we can verify that the topic has been gaining interest as it can be seen in Fig. 5, both in academic and grey literature data sources the interest on the topic rose considerably after 2017.

The year 2019 has less studies because this review only took into consideration the studies until the 10th of April of the same year.

Final selection of studies only contained 2 academic articles and much of the literature use to answer the research questions is based on Blogs and articles from industry professionals. Table 6 summarizes number of articles based on literature source.

Table 6. Final number of articles by literature source.

Literature source	Number of articles
Academic	2
Grey	11

6   Reporting the Review

This MLR phase presents the research done on DevSecOps to identify its metrics. We used Google Scholar, Google Search, IEEE Explore, Springer and ACM Library to locate literature and after applying our inclusion and exclusion criteria, 15 articles were found to be relevant to our search terms. Only 2 of those were academic research papers. The remaining 11 consisted of blogs and articles. Based on the literature review found e 9 relevant metrics were reported by professionals. Table 7 lists and describes identified metrics.

Table 7. DevSecOps metrics

Metric	References	Description	Goal	Measuring
Defect density	[17–20]	This metric can be defined has the number of confirmed defects detected in software/ component during a defined period of development/operation divided by the size of the software/component	Helps security teams and developers negotiate reasonable goals to reduce defect density over time	Defect density is measured by dividing the total number of confirmed defects by the total line of codes of all the modules in the new release. Ideal is to have the lowest density value possible
Defect burn rate	[17, 19, 21]	Indicates how quickly the team is addressing defects	Measuring development team productivity solving defects	Take the total number of defects found in development and divided it by the sum of defects found in development and production and multiplied by 100. If the rate has a high value it means the team is being effective

(continued)

Table 7. (*continued*)

Critical risk profiling	[17, 22–26]	Is the relation between issue criticality and the value of that vulnerability to possible attackers	The goal of this is metric is help prioritize the order development teams should address issues	Vulnerability should be associated with a score for a criticality and another that defines the value of that vulnerability to attackers. Vulnerabilities that have high score in both criticality and value should be handle first. Having vulnerabilities with low score on criticality and value is a good indicator
Top vulnerability types	[17, 20, 27]	Lists the top vulnerability types and the most recurring ones	Helps planning training provided to developers accordingly and capacitate them with knowledge to handle and mitigate returning vulnerabilities	Keeping track of most recurring vulnerabilities related with software development (example OWASP Top 10). A good indicator is to have the lowest number of vulnerabilities without a mitigation plan
Number of adversaries per application	[17, 26]	Identifies how many adversaries an application might have this metric is associated with the practice of Threat Modelling and Risk Analysis	The goal is to identify the applications inside an organization that are more exposed to possible attacks and prepare accordingly	Team exercise where the objective is to think how many adversaries they think an application as and register those findings
Adversary return rate	[17]	Measures how often an adversary will use the same strategy and procedures	Helps define appropriate training to better handle these attacks	Measure is done by counting the number of times adversaries use the same attacking strategy and compiling into a ranking that visible for every team member. Ideal is to have a plan to handle each attacking strategy
Point of risk per device	[18]	Tracks the number of vulnerabilities per server	Helps prioritize these vulnerabilities according to their criticality giving special attention to the ones that are most exposed to attack from the internet	Identify and keep track of unpatched vulnerabilities per server. The number of vulnerabilities should tend to zero

(*continued*)

Table 7. (*continued*)

Number of continuous delivery cycles per month	[18, 19, 21, 26]	Number of successful deploys to production per month	Measuring how quickly code changes can be deployed to production	This metric is measured by counting the number of attempts to deploy versus the number of successful attempts. A positive value is to have the highest number of successful attempts
Number of issues during red teaming drills	[21, 26]	Number of found issues and fixed by Red Team	Measuring Red Team Effectiveness	Measured by counting the number of defects found and fixed by the Red Team

7   Conclusion and Future Work

This MLR presents the research done on DevSecOps to identify metrics associated with DevSecOps that can be used to measure its effectiveness. DevSecOps is a recent topic has it was established earlier it is expected to continue to grow. It was very hard to find information regarding metrics associated with DevSecOps special in academic literature. Even so it was possible to identify a total 9 metrics as indicators of DevSecOps effectiveness. This topic is expected to grow and for that reason it's study should continue; this study serves as the initial support for further studies.

This study for academics may serve has the basis for further research into DevSecOps metrics or other related metrics. For Professionals this study summarizes the principal metrics for measuring DevSecOps effectiveness in one document.

Since DevSecOps is a trending topic and this study had an exploratory nature, further researches may continue the study performing interviews and surveys with DevSecOps professionals to tune and complement the proposed metrics as well as what is the outcome of each one. Plus, it would also be interesting to understand what mechanisms and policies could be implemented to mitigate the security issues that the presented metrics are intended to measure. The authors are already pursuing this investigation line.

References

1. Silva, M., Faustino, J., Pereira, R., Da Silva, M.M.: Productivity gains of DevOps adoption in an IT team: a case study. In: Designing Digitalization, Lund (2018)
2. Mohan, V., Othmane, L.B.: SecDevOps: is it a marketing buzzword? - mapping research on security in DevOps. In: 11th International Conference on Availability, Reliability and Security (ARES), Salzburg (2016)
3. Rahman, A.A.U., Williams, L.: Software security in DevOps: synthesizing practitioners perceptions and practices. In: International Workshop on Continuous Software Evolution and Delivery, New York (2016)
4. Bass, L., Holz, R., Rimba, P., Tran, A.B., Zhu, L.: Securing a deployment pipeline. In: Third International Workshop on Release Engineering, New Jersey (2015)

5. Myrbakken, H., Colomo-Palacios, R.: DevSecOps: a multivocal literature review. In: Mas, A., Mesquida, A., O'Connor, Rory V., Rout, T., Dorling, A. (eds.) SPICE 2017. CCIS, vol. 770, pp. 17–29. Springer, Cham (2017). https://doi.org/10.1007/978-3-319-67383-7_2

6. Fenton, N., Bieman, J.: Software Metrics. CRC Press, Boca Raton (2015)

7. Garousi, V., Michael Felderer, M., Mäntylä, M.V.: The need for multivocal literature reviews in software engineering: complementing systematic literature reviews with grey literature. In: 20th International Conference on Evaluation and Assessment in Software Engineering (EASE 2016), New York (2016)

8. Elmore, R.F.: Comment on "towards rigor in reviews of multivocal literatures: applying the exploratory case study method". Rev. Educ. Res. **61**, 293–297 (1991)

9. Smeds, J., Nybom, K., Porres, I.: DevOps: a definition and perceived adoption impediments. In: Lassenius, C., Dingsøyr, T., Paasivaara, M. (eds.) XP 2015. LNBIP, vol. 212, pp. 166–177. Springer, Cham (2015). https://doi.org/10.1007/978-3-319-18612-2_14

10. Roche, J.: Adopting DevOps practices in quality assurance. Commun. ACM **56**(11), 8–20 (2013)

11. Bang, S.K., Chung, S., Choh, Y., Dupuis, M.D.: A grounded theory analysis of modern web applications: knowledge, skills, and abilities for DevOps. In: 2nd Annual Conference on Research in Information Technology, New York (2013)

12. Lwakatare, L.E., Kuvaja, P., Oivo, M.: Dimensions of DevOps. In: Lassenius, C., Dingsøyr, T., Paasivaara, M. (eds.) XP 2015. LNBIP, vol. 212, pp. 212–217. Springer, Cham (2015). https://doi.org/10.1007/978-3-319-18612-2_19

13. Virmani, M.: Understanding DevOps & bridging the gap from continuous integration to continuous delivery. In: INTECH 2015, Pontevedra (2015)

14. Ebert, C., Gallardo, G., Hernantes, J., Serrano, N.: DevOps. IEEE Softw. **33**, 94–100 (2016)

15. Ray, H.T., Vemuri, R., Kantubhukta, H.R.: Toward an automated attack model for red teams. IEEE Secur. Privacy **3**(4), 18–25 (2005)

16. Kitchenham, B.: Procedures for Performing Systematic Reviews, Keele University Technical Report TR/SE-0401. Keele University, Keele (2004)

17. Chickowski, E.: Seven Winning DevSecOps Metrics Security Should Track, Bitdefender, 1 May 2018. https://businessinsights.bitdefender.com/seven-winning-devsecops-metrics-security-should-track. Accessed 25 Mar 2019

18. Humphrey, A.: Diving into DevSecOps: Measuring Effectiveness & Success, Armor, 16 January 2018. https://www.armor.com/blog/diving-devsecops-measuring-effectiveness-success/. Accessed 29 Mar 2019

19. Jerbi, A.: InfoWorld, 13 November 2017. https://www.infoworld.com/article/3237046/kpis-for-managing-and-optimizing-devsecops-success.html. Accessed 25 Mar 2019

20. Hsu, T.: Hands-On Security in DevOps. Pack Publishing, Birmingham (2018)

21. Crouch, A.: https://www.agileconnection.com. Agile Connection, 13 December 2017. https://www.agileconnection.com/article/devsecops-incorporate-security-devops-reduce-software-risk. Accessed 26 Mar 2019

22. Casey, K.: Enterprisers Project, 19 June 2018. https://enterprisersproject.com/article/2018/6/how-build-strong-devsecops-culture-5-tips?page=1. Accessed 26 Mar 2019

23. Woodward, S.: BrightTalk, 18 September 2018. https://www.brighttalk.com/webcast/499/333412/devsecops-metrics-approaches-in-2018. Accessed 27 Mar 2019

24. Vijayan, J.: TechBeacon. https://techbeacon.com/security/6-devsecops-best-practices-automate-early-often. Accessed 1 Apr 2019

25. Raynaud, F.: DevSecCon, June 2017. https://www.devseccon.com/wp-content/uploads/2017/07/DevSecOps-whitepaper.pdf. Accessed 31 Mar 2019

26. Paule, C.: Securing DevOps — Detection of Vulnerabilities in CD Pipelines. University of Stuttgart, Stuttgart (2018)

27. Jose, F.: Effective DevSecops, 3 July 2018. https://medium.com/@fabiojose/effective-devsecops-f22dd023c5cd. Accessed 3 Apr 2019
28. Rao, M.: Synopsys, 6 July 2017. https://www.synopsys.com/blogs/software-security/devsecops-pipeline-checklist/. Accessed 2 Apr 2019
29. Romeo, C.: Techbeacon, Microfocus. https://techbeacon.com/devops/3-most-crucial-security-behaviors-devsecops. Accessed 3 Mar 2019

Enculturation of Cyber Safety Awareness for Communities in South Africa

Dorothy Scholtz and Elmarie Kritzinger[✉]

University of South Africa, Pretoria, South Africa
{kritze, scholid}@unisa.ac.za

Abstract. The internet has become so integrated with users' daily activities, that cyber users interweave their daily activities automatically between the physical and cyberspace without noticing. Cyberspace can be referred to as a virtual computer world, which includes the connectivity of multiple networks. These connections between multiple networks within cyberspace form a global computer network to enable online communication between cyber users. Cyber users connect to cyberspace for socialising, work and educational purposes. The advantages of cyberspace are enormous and to a great benefit to all cyber users and cyber business. However, cyberspace opens the door to a number of possible cyber risks and cybercrimes that can affect cyber users. Cybercrimes and risks relate to either financial loss, disruption or damage to the reputation of a cyber user or organisation. These cybercrimes can include hacking, phishing or identity theft. Cyber users may not be aware of or knowledgeable regarding cyber risks and cybercrimes. The cyber user needs to be cyber safety conscious in order to be protected against cyber risks and cybercrimes. In many instances, cyber users within the industrial sector are being made aware of cyber risks through education and training programmes within their working environment. However, many cyber users within communities in South Africa are not working in industry and therefore do not have access to opportunities regarding cyber safety awareness. This research aims to investigate the level of cyber safety awareness within communities and propose a number of approaches that can be used to create and implement cyber-safety awareness programmes and material within different communities. Differently communities within South Africa have different needs that can range from different languages, learning approaches and community-defined processes and procedures. A quantitative research method and random sampling were used to obtain data about cyber safety awareness within communities. In the research, a survey with full ethical clearance was used.

Keywords: Cyber user · Cyber space · Cyber risks · Cybercrime · Cyber safety awareness · Communities · Peer to peer education · Cyber safety awareness programmes

1 Introduction

Cyberspace is the online world of the connection of computer networks including the internet. Cyberspace has changed the way cyber users are conducting their daily activities such as communicating, using social media, doing shopping and travelling

© Springer Nature Switzerland AG 2019
S. Wrycza and J. Maślankowski (Eds.): SIGSAND/PLAIS 2019, LNBIP 359, pp. 91–104, 2019.
https://doi.org/10.1007/978-3-030-29608-7_8

[1]. Using cyberspace to accomplish personal and work-related activities have become second nature to cyber users. Cyber users perform their daily activities automatically and without even paying attention to the how, where and when of completing it. Cyberspace has opened up opportunities for cyber users to such an extent that it has improved the cyber user's living standards tremendously. However, cyberspace can also expose cyber users to cyber risks and cybercrimes.

Cyber users are extremely vulnerable to a variety of cyber risks and cybercrimes; such as identity theft, cyber bullying, cyber stalking and phishing [2]. Cyber users may not be aware or educated regarding cyber risks and cybercrimes, leaving them vulnerable to these risks and crimes [1]. Cyber risks and cybercrimes can be executed by any cyber user in cyberspace with the intent to break the law; such cyber user is then called an offender [3]. Cyber users need cyber safety awareness to guide them against cyber risks and cybercrimes [1]. Cyber safety awareness can be introduced in a community to educate the community members, also known as cyber users to become aware of cyber safety. The aim of this research is to determine community-based factors (needs) that will enhance cyber safety awareness within communities. Each community is different with different needs and requirements. This research proposes a number of factors through a proposed framework that can be used to create cyber-safety awareness programmes and material for individual communities based on their needs.

2   Background

Cyberspace can be referred to as a virtual computer world; more specifically cyberspace is an electronic medium that is used to form a global computer network to enable online communication between people [4]. Cyber users are people who work or play in cyberspace, thus carrying out daily activities in cyberspace [4].

Routley had identified in the 2019 Global Risks Report, data fraud and theft and cyber-attacks to be in the top five likely cyber risks to occur in 2019 [5]. The Global Risks Perception Survey is conducted annually. The Global Risks Perception Survey looks at which risks are viewed by global decision-makers to be likely to increase in that specific year. According to the Global Risks Perception Survey for 2019, the following are likely to increase, namely cyber-attacks and personal identity theft [5]. Palmer also indicated in the report to the World Economic Forum that the following cyber risks, data breaches and cyber-attacks are among the top five global risks facing the world today [6].

The South African Banking Risk Information Centre (SABRIC) indicated that South Africa has the third highest number of cybercrime victims in the world; where about R2.2bn are lost annually to cyber-attacks [7]. Smith indicated that according to Cyber security company Kaspersky Lab, the cyber-attacks in South Africa increased by 22% in the first quarter of 2019 compared to the first quarter of 2018 [8]. Thus 13 842 attempted cyber-attacks in South Africa per day. This is an alarming increase in cyber-attacks for any country not only for South Africa and will have a huge impact on South Africa's economy.

Kemp indicates that according to the 2018 Global Digital Suite of Reports from We Are Social and Hootsuite, 53% of people worldwide are using the internet. Furthermore, the reports indicated that 51% of people in Southern Africa are internet users [9].

With the statistics given in the background section, it is important for the cyber user to realise that it is vital to be cyber safe. In the next section on cyber safety, we will elucidate the terms, cyber risks and cybercrimes.

2.1 Cyber Safety

Cyber safety is the safe and responsible use of information and communication technologies [10]. Cyber risks relate to either financial loss, disruption or damage to the reputation of a cyber user or organization [11]. Cybercrime is a crime where a computer is the object of the crime such as hacking, phishing or identity theft or the computer is used as a tool to commit an offence such as hate crimes [12].

The cyber risks and cybercrimes that will be discussed in this section are identity theft, cyber bullying, cyber stalking, phishing and online fraud (scams).

Identify theft, cyberstalking and online scams are identified by Betternet as the top cyber risks and cybercrimes [13]. The community members in the communities that were used in the study identified the other two cyber risks or cybercrimes as cyber bullying and phishing.

- Identity theft is the deliberate and unlawful use of a cyber user's identity; the offenders will then gain a financial advantage over the cyber user [14].
- Cyber bullying or online bullying is a form of bullying using social media sites. Cyber bullying behaviour is a repeated behaviour that can include the following: posting rumours, threats, sexual remarks or hate speech [15].
- Cyberstalking refers to the internet or any other electronic means used to stalk or harass another cyber user. Cyberstalking may include false accusations, defamation and slander [16].
- Phishing is a dishonest attempt to obtain personal information about a cyber user such as usernames, passwords and credit card details by sending out what seems to be a reliable electronic communication. The electronic communication can be in the form of an e-mail or instant messaging. The e-mail or instant messaging can then ask cyber users to go to a fake website and enter their personal information [17].

Online fraud (scams) refers to a cyber user willingly giving away money under false pretenses. An example of an online scam is charity fraud [13].

The cyber user can be exposed to or be involved with the cyber risks or cybercrimes that were identified in this section. The cyber user will then be a victim and can be harmed in the process. To prevent harm from befalling the cyber user, such user needs to be protected and be cyber safety aware [18].

2.2 Cyber Safety Awareness Amongst Cyber Users

Cyber users who are working in industry are exposed to cyber safety knowledge in the workplace. Unfortunately, cyber users who are not working have little or no exposure to cyber safety knowledge and therefore lack awareness of how to protect themselves and their information within cyberspace. It is therefore vital that all cyber users are made aware regarding cyber safety if they have not obtained such awareness within their working environment. It is important for cyber users outside of the industry sector to be cyber safety aware, because they need to be protected against cyber risk and cybercrime. Cyber users outside of the industry sector are normally the community, which includes children, parents and the elderly. These members of the community need to keep themselves and other cyber users in the community safe from cyber-crimes. Informing communities about cyber safety is important, because a larger group of cyber users can be communicated to simultaneously, thus protecting more cyber users by making them aware of cyber risks and cybercrimes. If one community is made aware, they can educate other communities thereby making more communities cyber safety aware.

According to Kahla, more than 2,200 data breaches and 53,000 cyber security incidents were reported during 2018 [19]. Mobile banking fraud involving cyber users cost South Africans more than R23 million in 2018 and online banking incidents cost South Africans nearly R90 million [19]. SABRIC CEO Kalyani Pillay indicated that cyber criminals would rather focus on individual cyber users than try to breach a bank's security systems, because cyber users are more vulnerable and easy to target. Pillay also points out that social engineering attacks remain the biggest cyber risk to South African cyber users [19]. Kahla also indicated that 71% of South African cyber users surveyed in 2018 were deceived by tech support scams [20].

2.3   Communities

The research investigated if it was possible to introduce cyber safety awareness pro-grammes in a community to educate community members, also known as cyber users to become cyber safety aware. A community can be defined as people who have the same beliefs, needs and interests and who share or live in the same environment [21].

Community Participation
The lack of cyber safety awareness and skills is a great concern in South African communities. The South African Government and industry provide cyber safety awareness and skills initiatives within our communities, meaning communities in South Africa. Gilbert reported on the Safer Internet Day 2018 where Google collaborated with the SA Film and Publications Board (FPB) and became involved to focus on protecting children online and to empower learners, educators and parents regarding safer use of the internet [22]. Other South African departments and organisations such as the Department of Justice and Constitutional Development [23], Internet Service Provi-ders' Association (*ISPA*, 1996) [24] and Cybercrime Organization [25] also provide cyber safety information to South African cyber users. However, most of the time only information regarding cyber safety are provided and if there were actual initiatives to introduce cyber safety to the communities it would just have been a once-off initiative. There are no long-term plans or policies and processes in place in South Africa to enforce cyber-safety awareness skills in communities [26]. We also do not see the South African Government and Industry doing any follow-ups on the cyber safety awareness skills programmes that they offered. The communities therefore do not

receive any continuous learning with regard to the cyber-safety awareness skills that were introduced to them during the cyber-safety awareness programmes. There is also no transfer of cyber-safety awareness knowledge to other communities or community members. Thus rendering the effort that was put into the cyber-safety awareness skills programme meaningless whether it was in the format of a poster, workshop, presentation or talk on cyber safety.

Possible Approach – Peer-to-peer Education

Peer-to-peer education (learning) is the educational practice where a learner interacts with other learners so that they learn from one another [27]. Peer-to-peer education is important because everyone, meaning every learner has the opportunity to contribute to the learning of other learners. All learners are equal in this process and no one acts as the main learner or expert. All learners can then learn from each other; learners can share knowledge as well as gain knowledge. The group of learners can make use of a variety of learning techniques, such as group discussions, presentations, diagrams and videos [27]. A peer educator or tutor assists with peer-to-peer learning, and the roles can be interchangeable between peer learners and tutor [28]. Damon and Phelps first recognised the peer-to-peer learning approach, which includes the following: peer tutoring, cooperative learning and peer collaboration [29]. Peer tutoring is when one participant, the tutor, instructs the other participant the learner. Cooperative learning is the division of participants or learners into small groups and each one has a role and contributes to the team. Peer collaboration refers to participants or learners who are all novice to the subject or learning area, solving challenges together or learning from one another.

Palmer and Blake indicated that according to a study by the company Degree, 55% of workers turned first to their peers for assistance. Peer-to-peer learning can thus be a powerful development tool [30]. Craft identified peer-to-peer learning as the most powerful tool in the workplace [31]. Craft further indicated that peer-to-peer learning saves time and resources. Peer-to-peer learning allows the company to maintain knowledge within the company and to identify where knowledge gaps exist [31].

If peer-to-peer learning can assist companies to improve learning, knowledge sharing, identifying knowledge gaps and saving time and resources, it would also be a very powerful tool for educating community members or cyber users, as they are also referred to. Therefore, if a peer-to-peer learning approach is employed, community members will have the chance to teach other community members about cyber safety. Knowledge transfer will take place and any knowledge that is not known to other community members can be addressed and taught with the assistance of peer-to-peer learning. This approach will also save time and resources such as money, the latter being a very scarce commodity within most communities. Many community members might be employees, which makes their time valuable since their work is their primary responsibility. If a resource such as a teacher/tutor/facilitator is needed, such resource will have to be paid for or community members might have to pay to take cyber-safety awareness classes. Furthermore, follow-ups can be done regarding the cyber-safety awareness knowledge transfer to ensure that the knowledge is being utilised and not forgotten. More updated cyber safety information can then also be transferred to other community members due to their proximity within the community. Community members would be committed to empowering themselves and other members of the community, as they will not only keep themselves safe from cyber risks and cyber-crimes but also the community of which they form part.

3 Methodology

A quantitative research method was used, where random sampling was used to obtain data from cyber users. In the research, a survey was used as the data-gathering tool. Ethical clearance was obtained from the University to use the data collected from the different communities. The sections in the survey were as follows: Biographical information about the cyber user, cyber-safety awareness information, communities and awareness material. In the section on biographical information the general biographical information such as age, gender, qualifications, access to and use of cellphone and internet were gathered. In the section on cyber safety awareness, information on cyber safety awareness of the cyber user was gathered. In the last section, information was gathered on the community of the cyber user and the awareness materials that can be used to guide cyber users. 10 Participants were used to assist in the data gathering. The 10 participants were closely related to the different communities. The participants from within the communities handed out 167 questionnaires. The 167 questionnaires were completed by the community members. 10 questionnaires were excluded from the analysis due to certain sections of the questionnaires being incomplete.

4 Data Analysis

This section will present the findings of the data collection to determine cyber-safety awareness situations within communities. Figure 1 depicts the ages of the participants.

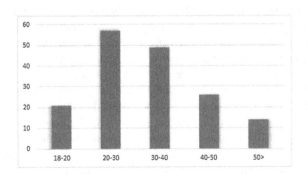

Fig. 1. Age representation of participants

The age participation indicated a bell curve of ages as depicted in Fig. 1. This bell curve verifies that the random sampling adhered to the dispersion of age groups through the different communities. The community participants were asked to indicate whether they had received any awareness, education or training regarding cyber safety awareness in light of their cellphone and internet use. Figure 2 depicts the cyber safety awareness received for the internet and cellphones.

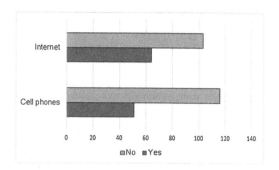

Fig. 2. Have you been informed about cyber threats relating to the internet and cellphones?

The data analysis indicates (Fig. 2) that more than 100 of the community partici-pants have not received any cyber-safety awareness information regarding the safe use (in light of cyber risk and cybercrime) of their cellphones and the internet. The follow-up question investigated whether community participants required additional cyber safety awareness and the results are depicted in Fig. 3.

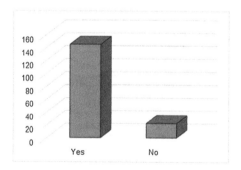

Fig. 3. Do you require additional cyber security awareness?

Figure 3 indicates that almost 89% of the community participants indicated that they require additional cyber safety awareness for themselves. The follow-up questions asked whether the participants thought that the community they are connected to are cyber safety aware and cyber safe. The results are depicted in Fig. 4.

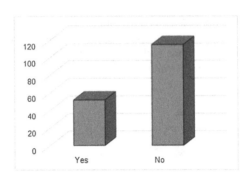

Fig. 4. Are your community cyber safety aware?

The findings indicated that 77% of the participants indicated that they thought their communities did not have the appropriate cyber safety awareness in order to protect themselves and their information. 100% of the participants agreed that their community would benefit from cyber-safety awareness training and education.

78% of the participants indicated that they would provide training in their communities after they have received the needed cyber safety knowledge, skills and awareness. The results form the basis of a peer-to-peer community approach. Members of the community transferring knowledge and skills to the rest of the community. The research also inquired whether community members would respond to cyber safety awareness if presented by community leaders and cyber victims as depicted in Fig. 5.

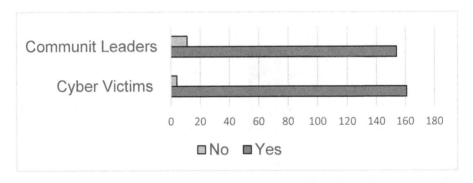

Fig. 5. Role-players in cyber safety within a community

In addition to the identification of role-players in Fig. 5, the following feedback from community participations were recorded:

- Awareness material should be realistic and relevant in relation to the community @hand, also fun and interesting
- Easily access to all awareness material

- Other languages (not only English)
- Accessibility and easy to use
- Take the literacy level of the community into account
- Follow up and support programmes
- The benefit to the community must be made clear
- Ensure that it is engaging with the targeted audience
- Clear and concise content of cyber safety material
- Real examples – relatable to the specific communities
- Improve training at schools
- Include in the school curriculum
- Elderly is often left out of the process
  - Internet service providers in collaboration with government
  - Focusing on the youth of the community.

5 Proposed Framework for Cyber Safety Awareness for Community Engagement

This section provides some guidance on how cyber-safety awareness material can be developed and integrated into the community to improve the cyber safety knowledge and skills of community members. This section takes into consideration that communities are unique and that different factors in terms of needs and cyber safety awareness must be considered. Factors such as mentoring, language and level of awareness have been identified. The following section will propose a framework and provide an example of how to ensure that the needs of communities are taken into consideration.

5.1 Framework

This research proposes a framework of elements that must be considered when designing cyber-safety awareness programmes for communities. Figure 6 indicates the proposed framework.

The proposed framework addressed the input of mentors and community leaders as part of the awareness process. Mentors are also an essential (derived from the data analysis) that must be included in the awareness process. The mentor will be responsible for the training of the community members by means of using the cyber safety programme. It would also be essential to have some of the victims identified within the community, so that the victims can also give input within the awareness programs. The community leaders also needs to receive cyber safety awareness training so that the community leaders can assist in the training of the community members. The proposed framework also includes the time span of cyber awareness programmes that should be

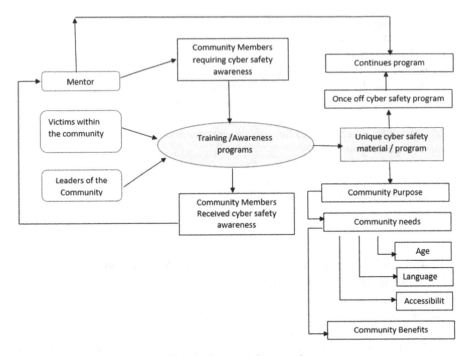

Fig. 6. Proposed framework

once off as well as an ongoing programme to improve cyber safety awareness. The community's needs are also important to include in the design of the cyber-safety awareness approach. The framework includes a few needs that were identified (derived from the data analysis). However, this list is not complete and can be added to depending on the communities involved. An example of one community factor, **language**, is addressed in the following section. At the end, the benefits of the cyber safety program within the community can be identified and the community leaders can establish if the community needs were covered.

5.2   Examples of Cyber-Safety Awareness Material for Communities

This section provides examples that were developed to address some of the issues raised by community participants.

It is vital that all communities have cyber-safety awareness material available in their chosen language. Figure 7 depicts the translation of one of the cyber-safety awareness workbooks that was created for communities.

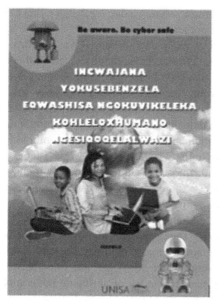 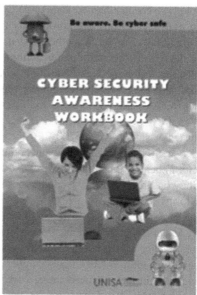

Fig. 7. Cyber safety workbooks in different languages

The English workbook in Fig. 7 was translated to IsiZulu, Afrikaans and Sesotho. The plan is to translate the workbook into all 11 official languages used in South Africa. It is vital that material is developed that is based on the needs of each individual community.

6 Conclusion

Cyberspace allows a cyber user to work or play, thus carrying out daily activities. The advantages of cyberspace are enormous and have great benefits for cyber users. However, the cyber user can simultaneously also be exposed to cyber risks and cybercrimes. Cyber users need to be cyber safety aware to be able to protect themselves against cyber risks and cybercrimes. Indications are that South Africa has the third highest number of cybercrime victims in the world. Thus, it is important to realise how vital it is to be cyber safe. Some cyber users are made aware of cyber risks and cybercrimes through their work environment, but other cyber users who are not employed or in a cyber-educated work environment are not so privileged.

The South African Government and Industry provide cyber-safety awareness skills programmes for cyber users within our communities, meaning communities in South Africa. However, most of the time, only information regarding cyber safety is provided and if there were programmes to introduce cyber safety to the communities, it was just once-off involvement. The research identified a possible learning approach, namely peer-to-peer learning to educate cyber users within the communities. Peer-to-peer learning will entitle those cyber users with knowledge regarding cyber safety where these cyber users can then educate other cyber users. Knowledge regarding cyber safety is then transferred from one community to another.

A quantitative research method was used to obtain data. A survey was employed to gather data from the participants within the identified communities. From the data analysis, the following was identified: more than 100 of the 157 participants have not received any cyber safety awareness regarding the safe use of cellphones and the internet. 89% of the participants indicated that their communities required additional cyber security awareness and 77% of the participants indicated that their communities are not cyber safety aware. 100% of the participants indicated that their communities would benefit from cyber-safety awareness training and education. 78% of the participants indicated that they themselves would provide training in their communities after they had received the needed cyber safety knowledge, skills and awareness. The result forms the basis of a peer-to-peer community approach.

The research proposes a framework that addresses the input of mentors and community leaders as part of the awareness process. The proposed framework also includes the time span of cyber-safety awareness programmes that should be once off as well as an ongoing programme to improve cyber safety awareness. A few identified needs are also included in the proposed framework. However, the list of needs are not complete and can be added to depending on the community. One need that the community identified was language. The research also introduced a workbook as cyber-safety awareness material. This same workbook has been translated into IsiZulu, Afrikaans and Sesotho. It is vital that material is developed that is based on the needs of each individual community, so that the community can be cyber safety aware and be protected against cyber risks and cybercrimes.

Acknowledgement. The cyber-safety awareness workbooks were created by Professor E Kritzinger that is also one of the authors of this paper.

References

1. Kortjan, N., Von Solms, R.: A conceptual framework for cyber-security awareness and education in SA. South African Comput. J. **52**, 29–41 (2014)
2. Kritzinger, E.: Growing a cyber-safety culture amongst school learners in South Africa through gaming. South African Comput. J. **29**, 16–35 (2017)
3. Broadhurst, R., Choo, K.-K.R.: Cybercrime and online safety in cyberspace. In: Routledge Handbook of International Criminology, pp. 153–165 (2011). Chap. 16
4. Fourkas, V.: What is cyberspace? March 2004, 123–153 (2011)
5. Nick, R.: Charts: visualizing the top global risks of 2019, 18 January 2019. https://www.visualcapitalist.com/top-global-risks-2019/. Accessed 14 May 2019
6. Danny, P.: Data breaches, cyberattacks are top global risks alongside natural disasters and climate change—ZDNet, 16 January 2019. https://www.zdnet.com/article/data-breaches-cyber-attacks-are-top-global-risks-alongside-natural-disasters-and-climate-change/. Accessed 14 May 2019
7. Shanice, N.: Cyber crime is advancing fast—Weekend Argus, 15 December 2018. https://www.iol.co.za/weekend-argus/news/cyber-crime-is-advancing-fast-18516412. Accessed 14 May 2019

8. Carin, S.: Mobile wallets a drawcard for cyber criminals – Kaspersky expert—Fin24, 2 May 2019. https://www.fin24.com/Companies/ICT/mobile-wallets-a-drawcard-for-cyber-criminals-kaspersky-expert-20190502-2. Accessed 20 May 2019

9. Simon, K.: Digital in 2018: World's internet users pass the 4 billion mark - We Are Social UK - Global Socially-Led Creative Agency, 30 January 2018. https://wearesocial.com/uk/blog/2018/01/global-digital-report-2018. Accessed 14 May 2019

10. Grey, A.: Cybersafety in early childhood education. Australas. J. Early Child. **36**(2), 77–81 (2019)

11. Saha, D., Mukhopadhyay, A., Sadhukhan, S.K., Chatterjee, S., Mahanti, A.: Cyber-risk decision models: to insure IT or not? Decis. Support Syst. **56**, 11–26 (2013)

12. Wall, D.: CYBERCRIME: what is it and what do we do about it? - Mapping out and policing cybercrimes (2011)

13. Betternet: The major types of cybercrime, 21 February 2018. https://www.betternet.co/blog/the-major-types-of-cybercrime/. Accessed 09 May 2019

14. Farina, K.A.: Cyber crime: identity theft. Int. Encycl. Soc. Behav. Sci. Second Ed. **5**, 633–637 (2015)

15. Cho, S., Lee, J.M.: Explaining physical, verbal, and social bullying among bullies, victims of bullying, and bully-victims: assessing the integrated approach between social control and lifestyles-routine activities theories. Child Youth Serv. Rev. **91**(February), 372–382 (2018)

16. Kircaburun, K., Jonason, P.K., Griffiths, M.D.: The dark tetrad traits and problematic social media use: the mediating role of cyberbullying and cyberstalking. Pers. Individ. Dif. **135** (June), 264–269 (2018)

17. Qabajeh, I., Thabtah, F., Chiclana, F.: A recent review of conventional vs. automated cybersecurity anti-phishing techniques. Comput. Sci. Rev. **29**, 44–55 (2018)

18. Strawser, B.J., Joy, D.J.: Cyber security and user responsibility: surprising normative differences. Procedia Manuf. **3**(Ahfe), 1101–1108 (2015)

19. Cheryl, K.: 2019: What to expect from cyber criminals, 30 November 2018. https://www.thesouthafrican.com/news/2019-expect-cyber-criminals/. Accessed 20 May 2019

20. Cheryl, K.: The top five scams that fooled South Africans in 2018, 28 December 2018. https://www.thesouthafrican.com/news/top-five-scams-fooled-south-africans-2018/. Accessed 24 May 2019

21. Aslin, H., Brown, V.: Towards whole of community engagement: a practical toolkit, pp. 1–146 (2004)

22. Paula, G.: SA embraces safer internet day—ITWeb, 6 February 2018. https://www.itweb.co.za/content/j5alrvQlPa1qpYQk. Accessed 25 May 2019

23. Department of Justice and Constitutional Development (2019). http://www.justice.gov.za/cybersafety/cybersafety.html. Accessed 25 May 2019

24. ISPA (1996). https://ispa.org.za/. Accessed 25 May 2019

25. Cybercrime Organization (2019). http://cybercrime.org.za/international-resources/. Accessed 25 May 2019

26. Sutherland, E.: Governance of cybersecurity – the case of South Africa. African J. Inf. Commun. **20**, 83–112 (2018)

27. Andrews, M., Manning, N.: Draft for consultation a guide to peer-to-peer learning (2016). https://www.effectiveinstitutions.org/media/The_EIP_P_to_P_Learning_Guide.pdf. Accessed 14 Feb 2018

28. Swapnali Gazulaa, P.P., McKennab, L., Cooper, S.: A systematic review of reciprocal peer tutoring within tertiary health profession educational programs. Heal. Prof. Educ. **3**(2), 64–78 (2016)

29. Damon, W., Phelps, E.: Critical distinctions among three methods of peer education. Int. J. Educ. Res. **13**, 9–19 (1989)

30. Kelly, P., David, B.: How to help your employees learn from each other, 8 November 2018. https://hbr.org/2018/11/how-to-help-your-employees-learn-from-each-other. Accessed 25 May 2019

31. LaMesha, C.: Peer-to-peer learning: the most powerful tool in the workplace » Community— GovLoop, 12 March 2018. https://www.govloop.com/community/blog/the-most-powerful-tool-in-the-workplace/. Accessed 25 May 2019

Privacy Concerns and Remedies in Mobile Recommender Systems (MRSs)

Ramandeep Kaur Sandhu$^{(\boxtimes)}$, Heinz Roland Weistroffer,
and Josephine Stanley-Brown

Virginia Commonwealth University, Richmond, USA
{Sandhurk2, hrweistr, stanleybrowjb}@vcu.edu

Abstract. A mobile recommender (or recommendation) system (MRS) is a
type of recommendation system that generates recommendations for mobile
users in a mobile Internet environment. An MRS collects users' information
through users' mobile devices via inbuilt sensors, installed mobile apps, running
applications, past records etc. Although collecting such data enables MRSs to
construct better user profiles and provide accurate recommendations, it also
infringes users' privacy. This study intends to provide a comprehensive review
of privacy concerns associated with data collection in MRSs. This study makes
three important contributions. First, it synthesizes the literature on sources of
data collection in MRSs. Second, it provides insights into privacy concerns
associated with data collection in MRSs. Third, it offers insights into how these
privacy issues can be addressed.

Keywords: Mobile recommender systems · Privacy · Collection ·
Control · Awareness

1 Introduction

The use of smart mobile devices and the rapid growth of the Internet and networking
infrastructure have led to the emergence of mobile recommender systems [29].
An MRS is a type of recommender system that generates recommendations for mobile
users in a mobile Internet environment [45]. An MRS alleviates the problem of
information overload in a mobile environment through the support of mobile devices.

The exclusive features of smart mobile devices, such as the ability to provide
services to mobile users wherever and whenever they need it (i.e., ubiquity) has
enabled MRSs to collect data related to users' transportation means, health, income,
mood, location etc. [33]. An MRS collects such information from inbuilt sensors in
mobile devices [16, 36], installed mobile apps on users' mobile devices [11], call logs,
contacts, emails stored in mobile devices [2, 49], and users' web browsing histories
[17, 46]. Although collecting such data enables MRSs to construct better user profiles
and provide accurate recommendations, it also violates users' privacy. Privacy violations in MRSs are more complex than in traditional recommender systems due to the
collection of users' sensitive information however, whenever, and wherever.

Various studies have raised privacy concerns related to data collection in MRSs. As
per our knowledge, none of the studies have provided a comprehensive review of

S. Wrycza and J. Maślankowski (Eds.): SIGSAND/PLAIS 2019, LNBIP 359, pp. 105–118, 2019.
https://doi.org/10.1007/978-3-030-29608-7_9

privacy concerns associated with data collection in MRSs. The study by Toch et al. [39] provided a literature review on privacy issues in recommender systems with the focus on three technologies: social networks, behavioral profiling, and location-based web services. The focus of that study was not on MRSs as such. The study by Ricci [33] conducted a literature review of major issues and opportunities of MRSs specifically with the focus on travel and tourism. The study by Liu et al. [25] provided a literature review of context aware MRSs. That study didn't focus on privacy concerns in MRSs.

Our study is intended to provide a comprehensive review of privacy concerns/issues associated with data collection in MRSs and how these concerns/issues can be resolved. To guide our exploration, we make use of the theoretical framework on dimensionality of Internet users' information privacy concerns (IPC) proposed by Malhotra et al. [26]. According to Malhotra et al., privacy concerns of Internet users center on three major dimensions: *collection, control,* and *awareness.* These three constructs offer a sound perspective in examining privacy concerns in MRSs, because according to Pimenidis et al. [29], MRSs utilize Internet, smartphones and networking infrastructures to collect users' personal information and preferences.

The focus of our study is to examine MRSs users' privacy concerns with respect to data collection. We thus want to answer the following research questions: *(1) What are the different sources of data collection in MRSs? (2) What are the privacy concerns associated with data collected in MRSs? (3). What are the different techniques and procedures that can be used to address these privacy concerns?*

Our study makes three important contributions. First, it synthesizes the literature on sources of data collection in MRSs. Second, it provides insights into privacy concerns associated with data collection in MRSs. Third, our study contributes to MRS literature by offering insights into how these privacy concerns can be addressed. From a theoretical perspective, researchers can use the findings of this study to assess and mitigate privacy risks associated with MRSs. From a practical perspective, our study can help IT practitioners to effectively address these privacy concerns and develop more trustworthy MRSs. The structure of the rest of this paper is as follows: The next section discusses the methodology used in conducting the literature review. Next, the major findings are presented: sources of data collection, privacy concerns with respect to data collection, and methods to mitigate these privacy concerns. The study concludes by summarizing the findings and discussing limitations and future work.

2 Methodology

We conducted a literature review of articles in the top journals in the fields of information systems, management, logistics, marketing, health care, education, etc. The articles were searched using databases such as: Google Scholar, EBSCOhost, IEEE Xplore, and Web of Science. The motivation behind searching in domains other than IS is that MRSs are extensively used in all these domains. Moreover, these different streams provide diverse views on privacy issues in MRSs.

We identified the initial set of articles using nine descriptors: "mobile", "smartphones", "personalization system", "interactive decision aid system", "recommender agent", "recommender system", "consumer centric", "one to one marketing", and "privacy concerns". The descriptors other than "mobile", "smartphone", and "privacy" were based on Li and Karahanna's [22] definition of recommender systems. A total of 94 articles were retrieved from using the above search terms. In the next phase, the relevancy of the articles was determined from the titles and abstracts of the articles. Lastly, the remaining articles were read in detail for further verification. Articles that didn't contribute towards answering our research question were excluded from the study. This resulted in 51 articles for our review.

3 Sources for Data Collection in MRSs

The objective of recommender systems is to provide recommendations of various products and services to the users based on user profiles and preferences [48]. MRSs create user profiles by collecting user information from the users as well as their mobile devices.

3.1 Data Collected from Users

MRSs require users to provide personal information such as user name, preferences, addresses, etc. to utilize the system. Similar to traditional recommender systems, MRSs also require users to explicitly state their personalized preferences, constraints, and needs [47], such as favorite news channel for recommending daily news stories [33], favorite music for recommending music [34, 42], tourism related destinations, and specified information related to sight-seeing spots such as parks, monuments, etc. [47].

3.2 Data Collected from Users' Mobile Devices

In addition to collecting the data from users, MRSs also collect data about the users from mobile apps [11, 23, 36], in-built sensors [3, 6, 16, 20, 34, 42, 44, 47], applications running on mobile devices such as emails or chat messages [2, 7], and past records [17, 18, 35, 46].

Mobile Apps. Mobile apps are accurate representations of users' interests and preferences. MRSs uses installed mobile apps to predict user interest and built user profiles without requiring the users to enter their preferences, hobbies etc. MRSs analyze which apps are installed on users' devices to extract the information such as: personality traits, demographics like gender, age, salary, life events, and religion, location, time, activities [11, 36]. These systems don't read any data from the app itself, rather it uses machine learning approaches to predict users' interest from snapshots of the mobile apps installed on users' devices [11].

Lin et al. [23] proposed an MRS that constructs user profiles based on the actions performed by a user on a normal hotel searching mobile app. This MRS records each and every gesture of the user, such as zoom in, zoom out, and time taken to read the review, on the hotel-searching app to record the user's behavior. The MRS uses this information to generate the user's interests and recommends hotels based on that. Frey et al. [11] proposed an MRS that uses description and details of the features of the installed mobile apps to generate predictors such as: personal interest and gender.

Sensors. Mobile phones have inbuilt sensors such as: accelerometer, gyroscope, camera, GPS, sound sensors, microphone, etc. MRSs use these sensors to extract various user related information such as: measure blood pressure volume (BPV), transport means detection [16], personal interests [44], and accelerometers for activity recognitions [6, 16].

GPS location data is used to detect available footpaths or streets to identify a user's means of transportation i.e., whether the user is travelling by bus, car, on foot, or is inside the building. In addition, GPS information is used to provide personalized advertisements, recommend places, events, routes etc. [20, 44]. Furthermore, geotagged photos and check-ins on users' mobile devices are used to predict users' preferences [20]. Barranco et al. [3] proposed a mobile tourism recommender system that uses GPS data to extract a user's speed and trajectory to propose interesting points of interest (POIs).

A mobile phone's accelerometer is used to detect four different transportation modes: idle, walking, vehicle, and cycling [16]. Wang et al. [42] proposed a music MRS that utilizes accelerometer and audio input from a user's mobile devices to detect the user's activities in real time, i.e., whether the user is working, studying, running, sleeping, walking, working, shopping etc. Based on the inferred activity, it plays suitable music automatically.

The inbuilt camera in the mobile device is used to detect a user's emotions. Rizk et al. [34] proposed an MRS that uses users' emotions to streamline music from online radio stations. This MRS uses camera and face detection techniques to capture users' face images and later apply emotion recognition techniques to capture users' emotions. Face detection techniques locate the face within the image, crop out the face, and locate the midpoint and calculate the distance between the eyes. This data is then sent to a server to perform emotion recognition.

Application Running on Mobile Devices. Mobile users normally have multiple applications running on their devices such as emails, messages, calendars, social network accounts, contacts, call logs etc. MRSs construct user profiles based on information retrieved from these applications. MRSs proposed by Baglioni et al. [2] and Davidson et al. [7] are the exemplars of such kind of MRSs. The MRS proposed by Baglioni et al. [2] uses call logs, short messages and contact lists to recommend new contacts to the users. Similarly, the MRS proposed by Davidson et al. uses the user's social media accounts such as Facebook and Twitter, short messages, email, and HTTP traffic, to determine whether the user is a student, executive, bachelor, sports buff, technophile, retiree, homemaker, etc., and make recommendations about summer vacations, courses, sports, dating apps, etc.

Past Records. MRSs also utilize users' past records such as web browsing history, purchasing history, including prices and brand value, to make recommendations. Roussos et al. [35] developed a mobile-based personalized grocery system named MyGrocer that utilizes a user's previous grocery history and price preferences to offer negotiated prices for products from different vendors. Yang et al. [46] proposed an

MRS that recommends vendors' web pages, including coupons and promotions, to interested customers. The system analyzes customers' browsing history, such as web pages visited and location to create users' profiles. It also maintains vendor profiles, such as name, address, and webpage link. The system then matches vendor and customer profiles to generate recommendations.

Kim et al. [18] proposed an MRS named buying-net that collects information related to items the customer purchased, the prices of the items, and its brand value to construct a user profile. Jiang et al. [17] also use web-browsing history to create user profiles. The MRS collects users' behavior information from their web-browsing records and utilizes a K-nearest neighbors (KNN) classification algorithm to classify users. Later it uses a matching algorithm to recommend friends based on users' behaviors.

4 Privacy Concerns with Respect to Data Collection in MRSs

Since a mobile device is normally owned by a single individual, the usage of a mobile device and the type of data collected from the mobile device can reasonably be assumed to represent a user's interests and daily activities. The more knowledge about a user's interest and daily activities is collected, the greater the possibility of a user's invasion of privacy [4]. A user's perceived risks of privacy invasion negatively impact the adoption of an MRS for personalization [45]. It becomes crucial to understand the nature of users' privacy concerns for the rapid adoption of MRSs.

This study adopted three constructs, namely *collection, control,* and *awareness,* used in the theoretical framework proposed by Malhotra et al. [26] on dimensionality of internet users' information privacy concerns as the basis to review MRS users' privacy concerns. *Collection* represents the degree to which an individual is concerned about the amount of personal information possessed by others relative to the benefits received. *Control* refers to whether an individual has control over the personal information as manifested by freedom to opt out or voice an opinion. *Awareness* represents the degree to which users are aware about the established conditions and actual practices [26].

4.1 Collection

There is always a trade-off between users' privacy concerns about the amount of personal information possessed by MRSs and the value of benefits received from recommendations generated by MRSs. This trade-off is referred to as privacy-personalization trade off [24, 44]. Different users' have different level of privacy and personalization concerns. Depending upon the level of privacy versus personalization preference, MRSs users' can be classified into three categories:

(a) *User with low privacy concerns but high personalization preference:* Such users provide any kind of information in exchange for highly personalized recommendations [31]. They don't set any privacy sensitive restrictions on their mobile devices [24].

(b) *User with intermediate privacy concerns and intermediate personalization preference:* Such users provide some information to MRSs to receive intermediate
personalized recommendations [31]. They set some privacy sensitive restrictions
on their mobile devices [24].

(c) *User with high privacy preference but low personalization preference:* Such users
prefer not to share any information to MRSs due to high privacy concerns [31].
They will set privacy sensitive restrictions on all the applications running on their
mobile devices. Examples of such users can be found in the studies conducted by
Gallego and Huecas [12], Roussos et al. [35], and Kim et al. [18]. The users in
these studies expressed their concerns about not using MRSs due to network wide
distribution of their personal information.

When users with intermediate and low privacy concerns share information, they
place a certain level of trust in MRSs. They provide their personal information to MRSs
with an expectation that MRSs will protect their private information and use the
information only for functional purposes [4, 46, 48]. But users' trust gets violated when
some MRSs use the users' information for commercial benefits such as personalized
advertisements [4, 44]. Users' privacy concerns with respect to collection are depicted
in Fig. 1.

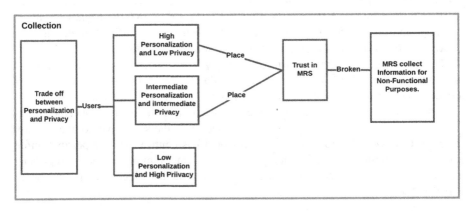

Fig. 1. Users' privacy concerns with respect to collection.

Collecting and utilizing users' data for commercial purposes such as personalized
advertisements not only results in violation of trust, but also in users' privacy exposures
[36], because the personalized advertisements are the accurate representation of users'
private and sensitive information such as marital status, income, etc. [27, 44]. This is
the type of information that some users would prefer not to share.

4.2 Control

MRSs set privacy policies in such a way that users no longer have full control over
their personal information. MRSs don't always consider consumers' privacy preferences or the issues that the users care about [32, 43]. Users are provided two options:

accept the privacy policy set by the MRS to use the system or reject the policy and not use the system [43]. By accepting the policies set by MRSs, users lose control over their personal information. Once a user accepts the policy, MRSs start collecting the user's information from different sources and construct and manage his/her profile in an ongoing basis [4]. And once the user's profile is generated, the personal information is analyzed, categorized, and acted upon by the MRS and other parties at any time, even when the user is not physically present [51].

Users have different levels of control with different MRSs. There are three types of MRSs: *Pull based, reactive,* and *proactive* MRSs [13]. A pull based MRS is a type of recommender system that uses overt mechanisms, i.e. the delivery of personalized content through user queries such as when users explicitly request lists of nearby points of interest. Reactive and proactive MRSs use covert mechanisms, i.e. the delivery of recommendations to users without their involvement. Reactive and proactive MRSs covertly extract users' behaviors through sensors enabled in users' mobile devices, purchasing histories etc. [13, 44] Users have some control over the pull based MRSs. These MRSs collect a user's information and provide recommendations only when the user submits the query. But users have no control over how these MRSs store and share data. In reactive and proactive MRSs, users have no control over their data collection as well as receiving recommendation [13].

Most MRSs use a server-side personalization approach to provide recommendations. Although this approach may be useful in dealing with issues like scalability, storage and computational powers, this approach at the same time prevents the users from exercising control over their data [1]. When MRSs use the server-side personalization approach, then users don't have the opportunity to decide who to share their data with, how to store their data, how to analyze their data and generate the recommendations, and how long to store their data.

Using the server side approach can expose a user's data to recipients other than the MRS, such as service providers (e.g. Google providing restaurant recommendations for nearby places), infrastructure providers (e.g. mobile phone company providers), law enforcement (e.g. police or other governmental agencies accessing service providers records) [28, 36], employers, and advertisers, etc. [40].

When users' data is stored on a server, there is also a possibility that the information is intercepted or abused (i.e., exploited for unintended or secondary usage) by hackers due to insecure transmission and storage techniques [28, 36, 38].

Although in general users prefer to have more personalized services [15], they also prefer keeping their personal information on their mobile devices rather than sharing it with MRSs [1]. Doing so enables them to have more control over their personal information [15]. Figure 2 depicts users' privacy concerns and issues with respect to control over their personal information.

4.3 Awareness

Awareness refers to the degree to which the users are aware about the established conditions and actual practices of MRSs, as well as consequences of sharing information with MRSs. MRSs disclose their established conditions and working practices in the form of privacy statements. Privacy statements detail data collection, sharing,

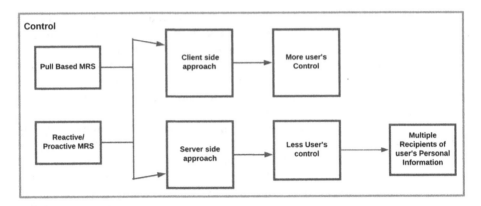

Fig. 2. Users' privacy concerns with respect to control over personal information in MRSs

and analysis policies and practices. These statements are often technical, vague, complex, and hard to read [32]. These statements are also not concise and are difficult for an average person to understand [4]. The technicality and complexity of these privacy statements prohibits users to fully understand and be aware of how much of their personal information is collected [50], how persistent the data are, who has access to their data, [4, 45], and how much information is disclosed/shared with other parties [19]. Moreover, the users may be travelling and may not have any incentive to read the privacy policies of the MRSs. So, users may end up giving their consent for data collection and its usage knowingly or unknowingly [4].

Individual factors such as level of knowledge [30, 41], digital competence [41], self-efficacy [21] and previous privacy invasion experience [44] also play a huge role in users' awareness of consequences of sharing their information with MRSs.

The level of knowledge refers to how much a user knows about the privacy risks associated with sharing the personal information. The level of digital competence refers to the skills, knowledge, and attitude that are required when using digital media to perform tasks, create and share content, collaborate, etc. [10]. The level of digital competence may depend upon age and generation [41]. Youths are more digitally competent than the older generations [33]. Individuals with high levels of knowledge and digital competence are better aware of negative consequences of sharing their private information with MRSs and more mindful in using the MRSs [41]. Most often, not all the users are technically proficient and knowledgeable to protect themselves from privacy infringements [28]. Users lacking digital competence and sufficient knowledge may end up giving excessive information to MRSs in exchange for highly personalized recommendations [37, 41], money, or gifts [30].

Self-efficacy represents the perception of an individual's ability to protect personal privacy. Individuals with higher self-efficacy have lower trust in MRSs and are better able to counteract the negative consequences of sharing their personal information [21].

Previous privacy invasion experience refers to past experience of personal information abuse. The individuals who have experienced privacy invasion in the past tend to be more aware of privacy risks associated with sharing the information with MRSs [44] and hesitate sharing personal information.

Users with low awareness often end up giving dangerous permissions to MRSs. These dangerous permissions can include allowing MRSs to access their contact information, messages, email, phone state, payment services etc. [50]. Giving such permissions enables MRSs to collect non-functional data. Collection and combination of non-functional data increases the context discoveries and potential privacy invasion risks. These risks are further exacerbated, when such data is shared with third parties [32]. Figure 3 depicts users' privacy concerns with respect to awareness in using MRSs.

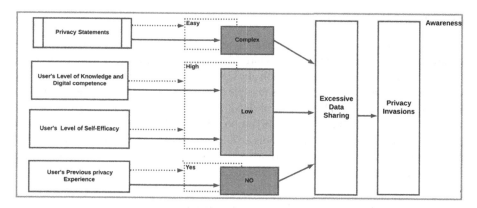

Fig. 3. Users' privacy concerns with respect to awareness

5 Methods to Mitigate Privacy Concerns in MRSs

This section details the methods proposed in the literature to address privacy concerns associated with MRS.

5.1 Limited Information Disclosure

User information disclosure can be limited in two ways: (1) Generalizing users' context information. Thus for example, instead of revealing that one is doing Pilates in Gold's gym, provide only more general information such as "exercising." (2) Giving users control to limit the amount of information stored on a server [14].

5.2 Use of Differential Privacy

Differential privacy allows data sharing without revealing an individual's identity. K-anonymity and L-diversity are two methods used in differential privacy. In the *K-anonymity* method, the information stored about a specific individual (i.e., information that includes quasi identifiers) is indistinguishable from at least k-1 individuals whose information is also stored in the MRS's central server. In the L-diversity approach, each quasi-identifier equivalence class has at least l represented sensitive attributes to prevent identification [41].

5.3   Incorporate Both Functionality and Privacy Preferences

In order to encourage users to adopt an MRS, it is very critical for the MRS to incorporate both interest-functionality interactions and privacy preferences in privacy policies to make personalized recommendations [24]. The privacy policies should also be concise and understandable in layman terms [4, 32]. MRSs should also inform the users about the kind of data collected and for what purpose. The users should be allowed to view their own data before it is passed on for analysis. Letting users see what data is collected, allows users to make informed decisions on whether to share it or not [5].

5.4   Client-Side Personalization

Instead of using a server-side personalization approach, MRSs can use a client-side personalization approach. The client-side approach refers to storing the user's information on the user's mobile devices. This approach allows users to exercise better control over their personal information. This approach is feasible due to increased computation and storage power of mobile devices [1]. Kim et al. [18], Sunanto et al. [38], Davidson et al. [7], Drosatos et al. [8], and Efraimidis et al. [9] proposed MRSs that store user collected data on the users' personal mobile devices. Doing so alleviates users concerns about the risk that their information may be intercepted or abused. In addition, a user's personal data can be anonymized at the device itself before sending it to the MRS [5].

5.5   Cryptography and Matching in Split Fashion

One way to avoid tracking the movement of users is to find overlaps among the users without having access to their full location tracks. There are two possible methods that can be used to avoid tracking: *cryptography* and *matching in split fashion*.

Cryptography allows matching seemingly meaningless properties that would only make sense to users, who would be the only ones able to translate the information back [36]. Homomorphic encryption, anonymity technology, and public key cryptosystem are the technologies used to preserve the privacy in mobile recommender systems. Additive homomorphic encryption has been used in the past to process user data and recommendations. Homomorphic encryption allows computation on ciphertexts without requiring to first decrypt the data. The outputs obtained from computation on cipher text matches the outputs of the operations, if they are performed on the raw data. Uploading the homomorphic encrypted data to a central server or using a third party to analyze the data mitigates the risk of privacy violations in MRSs [45].

The matching in split fashion approach allows users' personal mobile devices to extract some kind of aggregate measures and have the MRSs perform matching on these aggregate measures [36].

5.6   Value of Information (VOI) Metric

VOI metric is one technique that can be used to determine how much information is required to make recommendations and then to stop retrieving information from users or about the users once that level is reached [37].

5.7   Toggling Personal Information Refinement

The users should be given the option to toggle their personal information refinement. Doing so enables users to have more control over their data collection and personalization. When a user freezes his/her personal information refinement, the MRS stops tracking any additional behavior of the user, until personal information refinement and personalization is re-enabled [7].

6   Summary of Findings and Conclusion

This study found that MRSs collect users' data not only for functional purposes, but also for commercial purposes. Most MRSs store users' information on the server side i.e., on the MRS side. When the user's information is stored on the MRS's side, the user loses control over his/her personal information. Users often are not aware of what type of data is collected by the MRS and how it is utilized, stored and shared. Users are concerned that their personal information can be intercepted or abused.

In order to alleviate this problem, the user's information should be stored on the user's mobile device. This information can be encrypted before it is sent to the MRS, thereby allowing the user to have full control over data sharing and processing. The users should be allowed to toggle their personal information refinement and turn their personal information refinement on/off. When a user freezes his/her personal information refinement, the MRS should stop tracking any additional behavior of the user, until the personal information refinement and personalization is re-enabled. Moreover, the data should be anonymized/encrypted before it is sent to the MRS. The MRS can use homomorphic encryption to perform analysis on encrypted data. Homomorphic encryption allows computation on ciphertexts without requiring to first decrypt the data. The outputs obtained from computation on cipher text matches the outputs of the operations, if they had been performed on the raw data. Uploading the homomorphic encrypted data to a central server or using the third party to analyze the data mitigates the risk of privacy violations in the MRS.

In addition, the privacy policies set by MRS are not concise and are difficult for the average person to understand. These privacy policies don't consider consumers' privacy preferences or the issues that the users care about. Therefore, it is very important to set the privacy policies in such a way that they are concise, understandable and incorporate users' preferences. The MRS should also adopt some type of metric or technique to calculate how much data is required for generating accurate recommendations and at what level the data collection should be stopped. There should also be some rules/laws about how long the MRSs can store user's collected data.

This study provided a comprehensive review of MRS user's privacy concerns in data collection and the remedies for mitigating these privacy concerns. The findings of the study can help researchers and practitioners in assessing and mitigating privacy risks associated with MRSs and improve the likelihood of trustworthy mobile recommender systems development.

MRSs operate in three phases: data collection, recommendation generation, and recommendation display. This study focuses only on the privacy issues in the data collection phase. It doesn't include privacy issues in the recommendation generation and recommendation display. Future research can be conducted by conducting a literature review on privacy issues in the recommendation generation and recommendation display phases. Another limitation of this study is that it only included articles that were freely accessible and written in English.

References

1. Asif, M., Krogstie, J.: Research issues in personalization of mobile services. Int. J. Inf. Eng. Electron. Bus. **4**(4), 1–8 (2012)
2. Baglioni, E., et al.: A lightweight privacy preserving SMS-based recommendation system for mobile users. In: Proceedings of the Fourth ACM Conference on Recommender Systems, pp. 191–198. ACM, September 2010
3. Barranco, M.J., Noguera, J.M., Castro, J., Martínez, L.: A context-aware mobile recommender system based on location and trajectory. In: Casillas, J., Martínez-López, F., Corchado Rodríguez, J. (eds.) Management Intelligent Systems. AISC, vol. 171, pp. 153–162. Springer, Berlin (2012). https://doi.org/10.1007/978-3-642-30864-2_15
4. Beatrix Cleff, E.: Privacy issues in mobile advertising. Int. Rev. Law Comput. Technol. **21**(3), 225–236 (2007)
5. Beierle, F., et al.: Context data categories and privacy model for mobile data collection apps. Procedia Comput. Sci. **134**, 18–25 (2018)
6. Choudhury, T., et al.: The mobile sensing platform: an embedded activity recognition system. IEEE Pervasive Comput. **7**(2), 32–41 (2008)
7. Davidson, D., Fredrikson, M., Livshits, B.: MoRePriv: mobile OS support for application personalization and privacy. In: Proceedings of the 30th Annual Computer Security Applications Conference, pp. 236–245. ACM, December 2014
8. Drosatos, G., Efraimidis, P.S., Arampatzis, A., Stamatelatos, G., Athanasiadis, I.N.: Pythia: a privacy-enhanced personalized contextual suggestion system for tourism. In: 2015 IEEE 39th Annual Computer Software and Applications Conference, vol. 2, pp. 822–827. IEEE, July 2015
9. Efraimidis, P., Drosatos, G., Arampatzis, A., Stamatelatos, G., Athanasiadis, I.: A privacy-by-design contextual suggestion system for tourism. J. Sens. Actuator Netw. **5**(2), 10 (2016)
10. Ferrari, A.: Digital competence in practice: an analysis of frameworks (2012)
11. Frey, R., Wörner, D., Ilic, A.: Collaborative filtering on the blockchain: a secure recommender system for e-commerce (2016)
12. Gallego, D., Huecas, G.: An empirical case of a context-aware mobile recommender system in a banking environment. In: 2012 Third FTRA International Conference on Mobile, Ubiquitous, and Intelligent Computing, pp. 13–20. IEEE, June 2012
13. Gavalas, D., Kasapakis, V., Konstantopoulos, C., Mastakas, K., Pantziou, G.: A survey on mobile tourism recommender systems. In: 2013 Third International Conference on Communications and Information Technology (ICCIT), pp. 131–135. IEEE, June 2013
14. Hardt, M., Nath, S.: Privacy-aware personalization for mobile advertising. In: Proceedings of the 2012 ACM Conference on Computer and Communications Security, pp. 662–673. ACM, October 2012
15. Ho, S.Y., Kwok, S.H.: The attraction of personalized service for users in mobile commerce: an empirical study. ACM SIGecom Exch. **3**(4), 10–18 (2002)

16. Ilarri, S., Hermoso, R., Trillo-Lado, R., Rodríguez-Hernández, M.D.C.: A review of the role of sensors in mobile context-aware recommendation systems. Int. J. Distrib. Sens. Netw. **11**(11), 489264 (2015)

17. Jiang, W., Wang, R., Xu, Z., Huang, Y., Chang, S., Qin, Z.: PRUB: a privacy protection friend recommendation system based on user behavior. Math. Probl. Eng. **2016**, 1–12 (2016)

18. Kim, H.K., Kim, J.K., Ryu, Y.U.: Personalized recommendation over a customer network for ubiquitous shopping. IEEE Trans. Serv. Comput. **2**(2), 140–151 (2009)

19. Knijnenburg, B.P., Kobsa, A.: Making decisions about privacy: information disclosure in context-aware recommender systems. ACM Trans. Interact. Intell. Syst. (TiiS) **3**(3), 20 (2013)

20. Lathia, N.: The anatomy of mobile location-based recommender systems. In: Ricci, F., Rokach, L., Shapira, B. (eds.) Recommender Systems Handbook, pp. 493–510. Springer, Boston (2015). https://doi.org/10.1007/978-1-4899-7637-6_14

21. Lee, J.M., Rha, J.Y.: Personalization–privacy paradox and consumer conflict with the use of location-based mobile commerce. Comput. Hum. Behav. **63**, 453–462 (2016)

22. Li, S.S., Karahanna, E.: Online recommendation systems in a B2C E-commerce context: a review and future directions. J. Assoc. Inf. Syst. **16**(2), 72 (2015)

23. Lin, K.P., Lai, C.Y., Chen, P.C., Hwang, S.Y.: Personalized hotel recommendation using text mining and mobile browsing tracking. In: 2015 IEEE International Conference on Systems, Man, and Cybernetics, pp. 191–196. IEEE, October 2015

24. Liu, B., Kong, D., Cen, L., Gong, N.Z., Jin, H., Xiong, H.: Personalized mobile app recommendation: reconciling app functionality and user privacy preference. In: Proceedings of the Eighth ACM International Conference on Web Search and Data Mining, pp. 315–324. ACM, February 2015

25. Liu, Q., Ma, H., Chen, E., Xiong, H.: A survey of context-aware mobile recommendations. Int. J. Inf. Technol. Decis. Making **12**(01), 139–172 (2013)

26. Malhotra, N.K., Kim, S.S., Agarwal, J.: Internet users' information privacy concerns (IUIPC): The construct, the scale, and a causal model. Inf. Syst. Res. **15**(4), 336–355 (2004)

27. Meng, W., Ding, R., Chung, S.P., Han, S., Lee, W.: The price of free: privacy leakage in personalized mobile in-apps ads. In: NDSS, February 2016

28. Mettouris, C., Papadopoulos, G.A.: Ubiquitous recommender systems. Computing **96**(3), 223–257 (2014)

29. Pimenidis, E., Polatidis, N., Mouratidis, H.: Mobile recommender systems: identifying the major concepts. J. Inf. Sci. **45**(3), 387–397 (2019)

30. Polatidis, N., Georgiadis, C.K.: Mobile recommender systems: an overview of technologies and challenges. In: 2013 Second International Conference on Informatics & Applications (ICIA), pp. 282–287. IEEE, September 2013

31. Polatidis, N., Georgiadis, C.K.: Factors influencing the quality of the user experience in ubiquitous recommender systems. In: Streitz, N., Markopoulos, P. (eds.) DAPI 2014. LNCS, vol. 8530, pp. 369–379. Springer, Cham (2014). https://doi.org/10.1007/978-3-319-07788-8_35

32. Rasmussen, C., Dara, R.: Empowering users through privacy management recommender systems. In: 2014 IEEE Canada International Humanitarian Technology Conference-(IHTC), pp. 1–5. IEEE, June 2014

33. Ricci, F.: Mobile recommender systems. Inf. Technol. Tourism **12**(3), 205–231 (2010)

34. Rizk, Y., Safieddine, M., Matchoulian, D., Awad, M.: Face2Mus: a facial emotion based Internet radio tuner application. In: MELECON 2014 – 2014 17th IEEE Mediterranean Electrotechnical Conference, pp. 257–261. IEEE, April 2014

35. Roussos, G., et al.: A case study in pervasive retail. In: Proceedings of the 2nd International Workshop on Mobile Commerce, pp. 90–94. ACM, September 2002

36. Scipioni, M.P., Langheinrich, M.: I'm here! Privacy challenges in mobile location sharing. In: IWSSI/SPMU (2010)
37. "Tony" Lam, S.K., Frankowski, D., Riedl, J.: Do you trust your recommendations? an exploration of security and privacy issues in recommender systems. In: Müller, G. (ed.) ETRICS 2006. LNCS, vol. 3995, pp. 14–29. Springer, Heidelberg (2006). https://doi.org/10.1007/11766155_2
38. Sutanto, J., Palme, E., Tan, C.H., Phang, C.W.: Addressing the personalization-privacy paradox: an empirical assessment from a field experiment on smartphone users. MIS Q. **37**, 1141–1164 (2013)
39. Toch, E., Wang, Y., Cranor, L.F.: Personalization and privacy: a survey of privacy risks and remedies in personalization-based systems. User Model. User-Adap. Interact. **22**(1–2), 203–220 (2012)
40. Tsai, J.Y., Kelley, P.G., Cranor, L.F., Sadeh, N.: Location-sharing technologies: Privacy risks and controls. ISJLP **6**, 119 (2010)
41. Calero Valdez, A., Ziefle, M., Verbert, K., Felfernig, A., Holzinger, A.: Recommender systems for health informatics: state-of-the-art and future perspectives. In: Holzinger, A. (ed.) Machine Learning for Health Informatics. LNCS (LNAI), vol. 9605, pp. 391–414. Springer, Cham (2016). https://doi.org/10.1007/978-3-319-50478-0_20
42. Wang, X., Rosenblum, D., Wang, Y.: Context-aware mobile music recommendation for daily activities. In: Proceedings of the 20th ACM International Conference on Multimedia, pp. 99–108. ACM, October 2012
43. Xiao, L., Guo, F.P., Lu, Q.B.: Mobile personalized service recommender model based on sentiment analysis and privacy concern. Mob. Inf. Syst. **2018**, 1–13 (2018)
44. Xu, H., Luo, X.R., Carroll, J.M., Rosson, M.B.: The personalization privacy paradox: An exploratory study of decision-making process for location-aware marketing. Decis. Support Syst. **51**(1), 42–52 (2011)
45. Xu, K., Zhang, W., Yan, Z.: A privacy-preserving mobile application recommender system based on trust evaluation. J. Comput. Sci. **26**, 87–107 (2018)
46. Yang, W.S., Cheng, H.C., Dia, J.B.: A location-aware recommender system for mobile shopping environments. Expert Syst. Appl. **34**(1), 437–445 (2008)
47. Yu, C.-C., Chang, H.-P.: Personalized location-based recommendation services for tour planning in mobile tourism applications. In: Di Noia, T., Buccafurri, F. (eds.) EC-Web 2009. LNCS, vol. 5692, pp. 38–49. Springer, Heidelberg (2009). https://doi.org/10.1007/978-3-642-03964-5_5
48. Zhang, Z., Liu, K., Wang, W., Zhang, T., Lu, J.: A personalized recommender system for telecom products and services. In ICAART, no. 1, pp. 689–693 (2011)
49. Zhu, H., Xiong, H., Ge, Y., Chen, E.: Mobile app recommendations with security and privacy awareness. In: Proceedings of the 20th ACM SIGKDD International Conference on Knowledge Discovery and Data Mining, pp. 951–960. ACM, August 2014
50. Zhu, K., He, X., Xiang, B., Zhang, L., Pattavina, A.: How dangerous are your smartphones? App usage recommendation with privacy preserving. Mob. Inf. Syst. **2016**, 1–10 (2016)
51. Zwick, D., Dholakia, N.: Whose identity is it anyway? Consumer representation in the age of database marketing. J. Macromarketing **24**(1), 31–43 (2004)

Agile Methods and Software Engineering

Towards Agile Architecting: Proposing an Architectural Pathway Within an Industry 4.0 Project

Nuno Santos[1,2(✉)] 📵, Nuno Ferreira[2,3] 📵,
and Ricardo J. Machado[1,2] 📵

[1] CCG/ZGDV Institute, Guimarães, Portugal
nuno.santos@ccg.pt
[2] ALGORITMI Center, School of Engineering, Minho University,
Guimarães, Portugal
[3] i2S Insurance Knowledge S.A., Porto, Portugal

Abstract. Software architecture design, when performed in context of agile software development (ASD), sometimes referred as "agile architecting", promotes the emerging and incremental design of the architectural artifact, in a sense of avoiding "big design upfront" (BDUF). Performing "agile architecting" is not always straightforward, mainly because the architecture has a required life-cycle and each stage responds to different needs. There is a lack of a pathway that guides agile architecting in an end-to-end approach (from business requirements to deployment). This paper proposes a pathway that includes architecture design from software development life-cycle (SDLC) stages of software development that use ASD approaches, where two main artifacts are considered: a candidate logical architecture and a refined logical architecture. These artifacts are included in a pathway where they receive input from business processes perspective and guide software development during ASD iterations (Sprints).

Keywords: Agile architecting · Software architecture ·
Architecture viewpoints · Industry 4.0

1 Introduction

The role of architecture and architects have been changing due to the adoption of agile software development (ASD) approaches. Although an initial misconception because popular ASD frameworks (Scrum, XP, Kanban, DSDM) did not explicitly include architectural artifacts or roles, this role has been emerging towards a balanced design and implementation as the architecture emerges throughout the process. The architect plays a role in upfront planning, storyboarding and backlogs, sprints and working software stages of a project [1]. More recently, agile scaling frameworks, namely

This work has been supported by FCT – Fundação para a Ciência e Tecnologia within the Project Scope: UID/CEC/00319/2019.

S. Wrycza and J. Maślankowski (Eds.): SIGSAND/PLAIS 2019, LNBIP 359, pp. 121–136, 2019.
https://doi.org/10.1007/978-3-030-29608-7_10

SAFe, LeSS, DA 2.0 and EADAGP, have been adopted in industry, and architect's role have been specified by actively and passively support agile teams by driving architectural initiatives, participating in architectural runways, harmonizing governance requirements, and ensuring technical alignment in solution contexts [2].

One of the proposals for performing design as concepts and requirements emerge, included in the research of Abrahamsson [3] and Farhan [4], is the approach of a walking skeleton. Abrahamsson refers to it as an architectural prototype [3]. Farhan refers to it as a tiny implementation of the system that performs minimum functionality. Kazman proposes the design of a candidate architecture [5]. He defines this design as "start by quickly designing a candidate architecture even if it leaves out many details."

During a software development life-cycle (SDLC), the architecture aims different inputs, target-users and viewpoints at each stage. The rise of ASD approaches have been changing SDLC processes, which impacts on how architecture supports these stages. In these approaches, architecture design is sometimes referred to as "agile architecting". Agile architecting is characterized for performing design activities in a way that architecture and its requirements emerge throughout software development, where "big design upfront" (BDUF) is avoided because needs change and many features specified in BDUF are afterwards classified as "You Ain't Gonna Need It" (YAGNI).

This paper presents a pathway proposal for an agile architecting lifecycle (AAL), which analyzes the evolution of an architecture for a software initiative throughout SDLC stages, from an enterprise level to the deployment of software components. The AAL pathway has three main stages: Grooming, Backlog and Delivery. During these stages, the architecture evolves within different viewpoints, which are directly related between them (Concepts, Information Systems, Software Systems and Infrastructure).

This paper is structured as follows: Sect. 2 presents related researches in agile architecting and use of architecture methods within ASD; Sect. 3 presents the requirements for an AAL pathway and stage dependencies; Sect. 4 describes candidate and refined architecture using viewpoints; Sect. 5 demonstrates the pathway in a project; and Sect. 6 presents this work's conclusions and future work.

2 Related Work

2.1 Agile Architecting

Prause and Durdik argue that architectural design can be improved in agile methods by [6]: (1) agile architectural modelling using an incremental, customer-involved process; and (2) an initial vision of the system including initial design is created during the first iteration of the development, where architectural design is more a draft that is changed during later development; (3) more detailed design followed further on several iterations for designing the system; and (4) continuous iterative design where design is embedded into agile development and architectural artifacts are updated regularly.

The adoption of architecture methods implies its usage as a complementary approach to agile in the development life cycle, in parallel with up-front planning, storyboarding, sprint, and working software [1]. The architecture should emerge gradually sprint after sprint, as a result of successive small refactoring [3];

Performing lightweight amount of effort in up–front design, by using, for instance, a "predefined architecture" [7], walking skeleton [4] and simple artifacts (informal box-and-line diagrams, descriptions of a system metaphor, a succinct document capturing the relevant decisions, etc.) [8].

This way, the architecture is able to handle all the known "big rocks", i.e., requirements that are particularly hard to incorporate late in the project [9] and used as a starting point for the generation of User Stories to be incorporated in the Backlog artifact [10].

2.2   Architectures in Agile Software Development

Back in 2006, Kruchten, Obbick and Stafford stated the importance of architecture although when some perspectives only depicted its use in heavy documentation and Big Design Upfront (BDUF) efforts afterwards resulting in "*You Ain't Gonna Need It*" (YAGNI) features [11], which was later confirmed by Abrahamson, Babar and Kruchten that such was actually happening in many cases. [3]. the architecture should emerge gradually sprint after sprint, as a result of successive small refactoring [3]. It is more common that in agile contexts, architectural design is addressed by metaphors [12]. Barry Boehm balance the use of architecture and agility with risk management issues, by the amount of information available for planning [13]. A study performed by Yang, Lianga and Avgerioub showed that architecting activities performed within agile methods are [14]: Architectural Description, Architectural Evaluation, Architectural Understanding, Architectural Maintenance and Evolution, Architectural Analysis and Architectural Refactoring.

User stories in agile development relate primarily to functional requirements; this means that nonfunctional requirements can sometimes get completely ignored. Unfulfilled nonfunctional requirements can make an otherwise fully functioning system useless or risky. A main objective of integrating architectural approaches in agile processes is to enable software development teams to pay attention to both functional and nonfunctional requirements [3]. Like in any project, as the requirements are being developed and refined, they are inputs for the architecture design, and also allow identifying architecturally significant requirements (ASR). Alongside, more feature- or functional-oriented requirements are identified, as well as relationships between them and between the ASR's. They are further implemented in iterations based in their relationships. This way, the sometimes disregarded software infrastructure is considered at the same time as the features/functionalities within the ASD iterations [15].

Madison's approach [1], called agile architecture, advocates the coexistence of agile and architecture as complementary approaches by appropriately applying suitable combinations of architectural functions (such as communication, quality attributes, and design patterns) and architectural skills in the development life cycle (up-front planning, storyboarding, sprint, and working software). Literature shows other research works, namely presenting framework proposals that explore the relationship and synergies between architecture-centric design and analysis methods from the Software Engineering Institute (SEI) that regard architecture design and review within agile frameworks. Jeon et al. [16] propose a customized Quality Attribute Workshop (QAW) and Attribute–Driven Design (ADD) is used in Scrum projects, [4] uses Architecture Trade-off Analysis Method (ATAM) to validate architectures in a Crystal project, [17] propose an approach based in these previous mentioned works to use QAW, ADD, ATAM and Cost-Benefit Analysis Method (CBAM) within XP activities, and [18] propose a hybrid of QAW, ATAM and Active Review for Intermediate Designs (ARID) method for FDD. The Four Step Rule Set (4SRS) is used within the Agile Modeling for Logical Architectures (AMPLA) approach for deriving a candidate logical architecture and further incremental refinement [19].

3   Proposing an Agile Architecting Lifecycle

ASD frameworks typically are structured in three phases within the lifecycle: Stories (or Requirements), Planning (of the cycles) and Delivery (of a working software increment). Note that (continuous) integration sometimes fall inside Delivery phase (when continuous integration, continuous delivery and DevOps practices are adopted), otherwise the process includes a Maintenance or Operations phase. For instance, well-known ASD framework as Scrum includes the Stories definition within the Pregame phase [20], whereas eXtreme Programming (XP) lifecycle includes User Stories definition within the Exploration phase [12]. Planning – namely, the definition of the Product Backlog and its items – is also performed in the Pregame phase of Scrum [20] but in XP it is performed in the Planning phase [12]. Delivery of software is performed in the Development phase of Scrum [20] and Iterations to Release phase of XP [12]. The Postgame phase of Scrum and Productionizing phase of Scrum may be included in the Delivery phase of the development lifecycle, or in an afterwards Operations phase.

With that in mind, an agile architecting lifecycle (AAL) should be oriented to these three phases. We propose in this paper architecting tasks, artefacts, possible inputs and outputs, for each of the three phases: Grooming, Backlog and Delivery.

AAL should first propose a high-level architecture, composed by main functional requirements and that allowed defining a separation of concerns. This separation is input for planning of each concern implementation, which each relate to a subsystem of the architecture. During delivery cycles (e.g., Scrum Sprints), each subsystem is refined into a more detailed architecture, composed with logical components that at this phase have more detail for being passed on to implementation teams.

Approaches differ from using a predefined artifact to using simplified versions initially, but the approaches in [3–5, 7–9, 21–24] all advocate an initial model that afterwards is refined. Table 1 compares the research works presented in Sect. 2.2, within the proposed AAL phases.

Table 1. Comparison of agile architecting approaches and their contextualization within the architecting lifecycle

AAL phase	[17]	[16]	[4]	[25]	[18]	[1]	[10]	[26]
Grooming	Planning and stories	Planning and stories		Planning and stories	Develop an Overall Model, Build a Features List, Plan by Feature	up-front planning, storyboarding	Stories	Software Product Line (SPL) Backlog, Agile Product Line Architecting (APLA)
Backlog	Designing	Designing			Design by Feature	sprint	4SRS	Sprints
Delivery	Analysis and Testing		Analysis and Testing		Build by Feature	working software		Working Product-Line Architecture (PLA), Working Products (SPL)

In any SDLC, whether waterfall, ASD, or other, the performed software engineering disciplines typically fall under the scope of business modeling, requirements, design, implementation, testing and deployment. The difference between these SDLC relies in the time where they are performed, but inputs from all disciplines are required.

Based in this premise, AAL pathway includes all disciplines, with the goal of incrementally evolving an architecture and reducing BDUF. Figure 1 proposes including in an AAL pathway description of Context, Functionalities, a Candidate Architecture and, then, a Refined Architecture.

In terms of Context, it relates to the knowledge acquisition of domain and enterprise settings where software solutions will execute. The understanding of such knowledge is the starting point. Functionalities relate to the definition of software needs (in opposition to a more process and business orientation of the previous stage), e.g., the definition of a "minimum viable product" (MVP). Then, a first candidate version is proposed and refined afterwards in order to emerge during delivery cycles. Proposing a candidate version relates to defining a high-level architecture, composed by main functional requirements and that allow defining a separation of concerns. This separation is input for planning of each concern implementation, which each relate to a subsystem of the architecture. During delivery cycles (e.g., Scrum Sprints), each subsystem is refined into a more detailed architecture, composed with logical components that at this phase have more detail for being passed on to implementation teams.

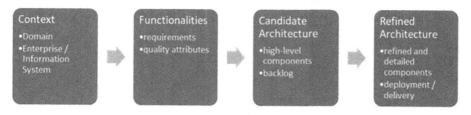

Fig. 1. Steps proposal for agile architecting

As referred, Context relates to knowledge acquisition of the domain, enterprise, business and information system where the project is scoped. It is composed in its majority with Business Modeling tasks. Typical examples of this exercise may be the modeling of the enterprise's business processes (*e.g.*, using Business Process Modeling Notation – BPMN), identification of technical and/or product glossary, relationships between main domain concepts, specification of the structure of the involved systems (like the name, the exchanged data, the data location – *e.g.*, which table from the database, etc.) and how to access that data. This is typically performed under an "as-is" analysis, however, even when the aim is to perform the characterization of the "*to-be*" situation, it is advisable that the SDLC firstly includes a proper domain characterization, by analyzing the business processes, the information (data), and the systems (hardware/software) that compose the ecosystem.

Additionally, in Functionalities, process reference models have an interesting role in requirements elicitation. For instance, it is common that manufacturing sector follows Supply Chain Operations Reference (SCOR). These reference models are composed with processes, sub-processes, roles, tasks, operations, that easily may be mapped in a business process notation language [27]. It is not expected that an enterprise follows only one reference model. For instance, the GS1 global standard for traceability is widely adopted for carrying out tasks for product traceability [28], and may be adopted complementary.

Now that the solution needs are identified – and properly specified – the next step typically relates to designing the system. System design is typically performed using a model, *e.g.*, an architecture. However, architecture design should be addressed as an iterative process, as design should start in a conceptual level and refined until it is detailed enough, which is to say the abstraction level goes from high to low during this process. For that reason, the pathway proposes designing a Candidate Architecture and afterwards a Refined Architecture.

Architecture design includes from conceptual level to more refined one [29]. Such argument is in line with the design process proposed by Douglass: architectural, mechanistic, and detailed [30]. Architectural design defines the strategic decisions that affect most or all the software components, such as concurrency model and the distribution of components across processor nodes. Mechanistic design elaborates individual collaborations by adding "glue" objects to bind the mechanism together and optimize its functionality. Such objects include containers, iterators, and smart pointers. Detailed design defines the internal structure and behavior of individual classes. This includes internal data structuring and algorithm details.

For describing the proposed logical architectures, candidate and refined, they are classified using a 3-layer schema based in the project lifecycle phase, MDA-based abstraction level, and Kruchten's 4+1 model views. The schema is depicted in Fig. 2.

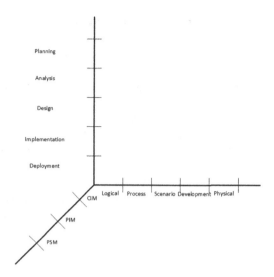

Fig. 2. Three-layer classification schema

Figure 3 presents the results from classifying Candidate and Refined architectures using the proposed framework. The presented classification is as follows:

Candidate Logical – **Phase**: Analysis/Design; **4+1**: Logical; **Abstraction**: CIM/PIM.
Refined Logical – **Phase**: Design; **4+1**: Logical; **Abstraction**: PIM/PSM.

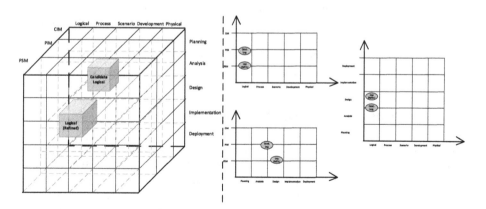

Fig. 3. Classification of Candidate and Refined logical architectures

4 Architecture Viewpoints and Definitions

An architecture has a particular scope. It may relate from software, hardware, organization or information, the overall system which encompasses all four, or the enterprise that hosts the system (or will host a future system to be developed). [31]. Within an organization or development project, many architectural viewpoints are defined, each more suitable for a given user but all related to each other. The "4+1" View Model [32] is one of the widely known architecture model, which presents the logical, process, physical, development and scenarios views. Other views like Siemens' Five-view Model [33], NIST Enterprise Architecture Model [34] or the *Zachman Framework*™ [35] present relations between these viewpoints.

In this paper, we propose the following eleven viewpoints, grouped in categories of Concepts, Information Systems, Software Systems and Infrastructure (Table 2):

Table 2. Architecture viewpoints categories

Concepts	Inf. systems	Software systems	Infrastructure
Conceptual architecture	Enterprise architecture	Logical architecture	Deployment architecture
	Process architecture	Component architecture	
Reference architecture	Information system architecture	Data models/Classes	Physical architecture
		Technical architecture	

ASD frameworks typically are structured in three phases within the lifecycle: Stories (or Requirements), Planning (of the cycles) and Delivery (of a working software increment). Note that (continuous) integration sometimes fall inside Delivery phase (when continuous integration, continuous delivery and DevOps practices are adopted), otherwise the process includes a Maintenance or Operations phase. With that in mind, an agile architecting lifecycle (AAL) should be oriented to these three phases. We propose in this paper architecting tasks, artefacts, possible inputs and outputs, for each of the three phases: Stories, Planning and Delivery (Fig. 4 and Table 3).

5 Demonstration Case: The UH4SP Project

In this section, a demonstration of the AAL pathway is described by presenting some modeling outputs from an Industry 4.0 research project called Unified Hub for Smart Plants (UH4SP). The UH4SP project aims developing a platform for integrating data from distributed industrial unit plants, allowing the use of the production data between plants, suppliers, forwarders and clients. The consortium was composed with five different entities for software development where each had specific expected contributes, from cloud architectures to industrial software services and mobile applications. The solution is based in the IoT, fog and cloud computing technologies.

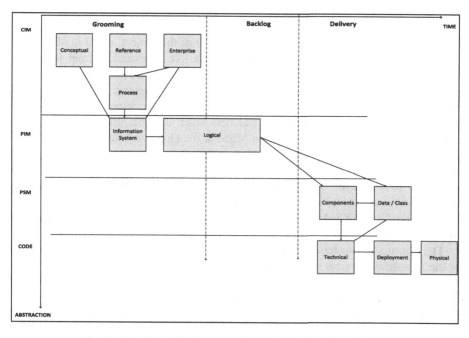

Fig. 4. Architectural views and abstraction within AAL phases

Table 3. The inputs and outputs of AAL artefacts

View	Input	Output	Relation SA
Conceptual	Product Vision, Domain model	Concepts, vocabulary, ontology	Information System
Reference	Process Reference Models	Domain's best practices	Process
Enterprise	Structure of Enterprise	Enterprise processes	Process
Process	Business processes, Process reference models	Process requirements	Information Systems
Information System	Process requirements, IT architecture	Information System requirements	Logical
Logical	Functional Requirements	Software requirements	Components, Data/Class
Components	Software requirements	Architecture requirements	Technical
Data/Class	Software requirements	Classes and methods	Technical
Technical	Software requirements	Detailed architecture requirements	Deployment
Deployment	Environment requirements	Deployment requirements	Physical
Physical	Infrastructure requirements-	Hardware	

5.1 Grooming

The Conceptual architecture, due to the I4.0 nature of the project, relied in identifying concerns aligned with Industrial reference models like Industrial Internet Reference Architecture (IIRA) and *Industrie 4.0* Reference Architecture Model (RAMI 4.0). By analyzing its layers, for instance within IIRA, the management of corporate-level production, tools for collaborative processes within the supply chain and the microservices architecture refer to the Business layer, and the production data at the industrial unit level are acquired from a MES, at the Operations layer.

This separation reflected the intended adoption of layers relating to business management, intermediate management at a cloud layer, and industrial local management at an edge layer. Such adoption was reflected in terms of the reference models for the Reference Architecture, by adopting NIST Cloud Computing Reference Architecture (NIST-CCRA) for the cloud layer and OpenFog Reference Architecture for the edge layer.

The information system architecture (Fig. 5) is thus based in the same separation. At the industrial physical space level (D), operations take place and the interaction between the various actors and the system is verified through the various interface devices. It is at this level that operational information is generated to support the services to be made available by the system. At an intermediate level (C), typically located at the edges for each industrial unit, distributed capabilities, namely related to computation, networking, and storage and offered. At the cloud level (B), a service-oriented architecture is deployed to support horizontal functionality integration. Finally, at the top-level (A), business apps, either desktop web apps or mobile web apps, are the main interfaces with human actors. They use the cloud services to execute their processes.

For the logical architecture design, the functional requirements for supporting the business processes under the information system were elicited, since a logical architecture is an abstracted view of a system supporting functional requirements. The requirements analysis in the UH4SP project included gathering the requirements from a set of "to-be" scenarios and model a set of functional decomposed UML use cases. The Use Case model was composed by 37 use cases. After executing an architecture design method that uses as input the Use Cases, the logical architecture (Fig. 6) was derived with 77 architectural components, grouped into five major packages, namely [36]: *P1 Configurations*; *P2 Monitoring*; *P3 Business management*; *P4 UH4SP integration*; *P5 UH4SP fog data*. The logical architecture diagram was then used to specify microservices, responsible for retrieving production data from local industrial units.

5.2 Backlog

The logical architecture depicts the organization of components, thus it provides the required functional behavior of the system. Based in that functional behavior, the necessary backlog of the required implementation work is defined.

Following a typical ASD backlog, the specifications about the software design, like the architectural components, were input for defining the backlog items, like user stories, their 'definition of done' and the acceptance criteria. Table 4 depicts a subset of

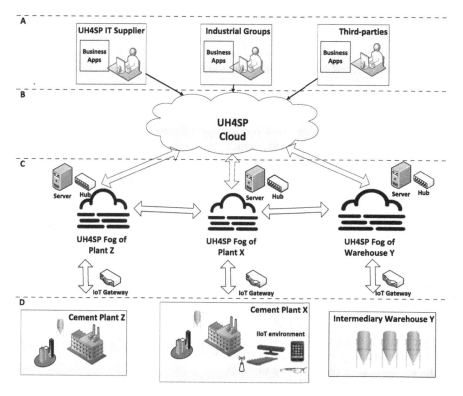

Fig. 5. UH4SP information systems architecture ([36, 37])

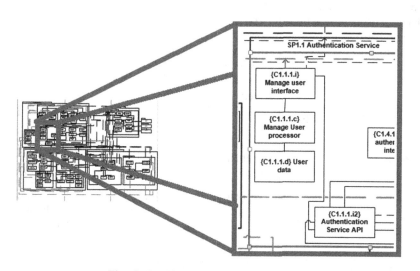

Fig. 6. UH4SP logical architecture ([38])

the backlog, where the defined user stories and acceptance criteria were defined. For traceability purposes, and for assisting in depicting the functionalities' behavior, the user stories are grouped by use cases and from the architectural components, based on the architectural method referred in the previous section.

5.3 Delivery

Having established the backlog, the UH4SP project began its implementation in Scrum Sprints. The backlog was refined, which reflected in increasing the details of

Table 4. Traceability between use cases and user stories from the generated product backlog, and from the use cases and components

Authentication Service			Use Case	Component
Use Case: {U1.1.1} Create user account			{U1.1.1} Create user account	{C1.1.1.d} User data
User Story	**Acceptance Criteria**			{C1.1.1.i} Create user interface
{US1.1.1.I.} As a System Administrator, I want to create a user account in order to configure user accounts.	{AC1.1.1.I.} System Administrator is able to create user			
{US1.1.1.II.} As a System Administrator, I want to change a user account in order to configure user accounts.	Acceptance Criteria: {AC1.1.1.II.} System Administrator changed user information is stored.			
Use Case: {U1.1.2} Edit user account				
User Story		Acceptance Criteria	{U1.1.2} Edit user account	{C1.1.1.d} User data
User Story	{US1.1.2.I.} As a System Administrator, I want to create a user account in order to configure user accounts.	Acceptance Criteria: {AC1.1.2.I.} System Administrator is able to create user	...	{C1.1.2.i} Edit user interface
	...	...	...	...

implementation needs of the components towards a technical architecture, like the issues from a framework development like .NET CORE, the data model supported by a MySQL server or the component's ports for communication purposes, namely using MQTT brokers.

Finally, within the Sprints, the deployment of the functionalities were also addressed. For that reason, the Deployment Architecture depicts the deployment location of the applications. The deployment architecture for the UH4SP project is depicted in Fig. 7: (a) UH4SP business apps layer, either desktop web apps or mobile web apps, are the main interfaces with human actors; (b) UH4SP integration layer, located at the edges for each industrial unit, distributed capabilities, namely related to computation, networking, and storage; (c) UH4SP cloud services layer, a microservice-oriented architecture; and (d) local industrial unit system layer, where operational information is generated.

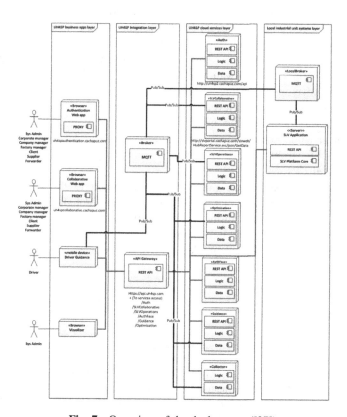

Fig. 7. Overview of the deployment ([37])

6 Conclusions and Future Work

Using ASD methods has led to the adoption of SDLC approaches that flavor the emergence of functionalities and architecture rather than performing BDUF that lead to developing YAGNI features. However, the emergence of new paradigms like Cloud Computing and more recently Industry 4.0, Internet of Things (IoT), machine-to-machine, cyber-physical systems, etc.) has led to companies often striving to properly elicit functionalities and design solutions, as their references and standards are still recent and immature so that companies may easily design solutions based upon them. This paper proposes an AAL pathway where software design evolves from architectural, mechanistic, and detailed design to development and deployment. The AAL pathway goes through three stages: Grooming, Backlog and Delivery. Throughout the stages, the architecture is designed under eleven viewpoints, grouped in categories of Concepts, Information Systems, Software Systems and Infrastructure. The viewpoints are more suited depending on the stage they are performed.

Grooming encompasses most architecture design. Starting from understanding the problem domain and existing references, the architect is able to specify functionalities and design a logical architecture. This logical architecture then allows defining a Backlog which scopes the software development in an ASD manner. As software increments are developed and the architecture emerges, the Delivery stage encompasses design at the deployment level. By using an Industry 4.0 research project called UH4SP, AAL was demonstrated using recent and immature references to start a software project with. Additionally, architecture design was supported throughout an entire agile SDLC, from domain and requirements analysis level and ending at the deployment level.

This research has still some points to be addressed in the future. The AAL described in this paper showed that architecture evolves throughout the SDLC and is supported by the viewpoints during such transition. However, there is space for approaches that automate such transitions. For that reason, we acknowledge that transition from design to technical and deployment (in Delivery stage) lacks of a proper transition support.

References

1. Madison, J.: Agile architecture interactions. IEEE Softw. **27**, 41–48 (2010). https://doi.org/10.1109/MS.2010.35
2. Uludag, O., Kleehaus, M., Xu, X., Matthes, F.: Investigating the role of architects in scaling agile frameworks. In: 21st International Enterprise Distributed Object Computing Conference (EDOC), pp. 123–132. IEEE (2017). https://doi.org/10.1109/EDOC.2017.25
3. Abrahamsson, P., Babar, M.A., Kruchten, P.: Agility and architecture: can they coexist? IEEE Softw. **27**, 16–22 (2010). https://doi.org/10.1109/MS.2010.36
4. Farhan, S., Tauseef, H., Fahiem, M.A.: Adding agility to architecture tradeoff analysis method for mapping on crystal. In: WRI World Congress on Software Engineering (WCSE), pp. 121–125. IEEE (2009). https://doi.org/10.1109/WCSE.2009.405

5. Kazman, R.: Foreword - bringing the two together: agile architecting or architecting for agile? In: Agile Software Architecture: Aligning Agile Processes and Software Architectures, pp. xxix–xxx (2013). https://doi.org/10.1016/C2012-0-01208-2

6. Prause, C.R., Durdik, Z.: Architectural design and documentation: waste in agile development? In: International Conference on Software and System Process (ICSSP), pp. 130–134. IEEE (2012). https://doi.org/10.1109/ICSSP.2012.6225956

7. Waterman, M., Noble, J., Allan, G.: How much architecture? Reducing the up-front effort. In: AGILE India, pp. 56–59. IEEE (2012). https://doi.org/10.1109/AgileIndia.2012.11

8. Erdogmus, H.: Architecture meets agility. IEEE Softw. **26**, 2–4 (2009). https://doi.org/10.1109/MS.2009.121

9. Cockburn, A.: Agile software development: the cooperative game. Pearson Education, London (2006)

10. Costa, N., Santos, N., Ferreira, N., Machado, R.J.: Delivering user stories for implementing logical software architectures by multiple scrum teams. In: Murgante, B., et al. (eds.) ICCSA 2014. LNCS, vol. 8581, pp. 747–762. Springer, Cham (2014). https://doi.org/10.1007/978-3-319-09150-1_55

11. Kruchten, P., Obbink, H., Stafford, J.: The past, present, and future for software architecture. IEEE Softw. **23**, 22–30 (2006). https://doi.org/10.1109/MS.2006.59

12. Beck, K., Andres, C.: Extreme Programming Explained: Embrace Change. Addison-Wesley Professional, Boston (2004)

13. Boehm, B.: Get ready for agile methods, with care. Computer **35**, 64–69 (2002). https://doi.org/10.1109/2.976920

14. Yang, C., Liang, P., Avgeriou, P.: A systematic mapping study on the combination of software architecture and agile development. J. Syst. Softw. **111**, 157–184 (2016). https://doi.org/10.1016/j.jss.2015.09.028

15. Bellomo, S., Kruchten, P., Nord, R., Ozkaya, I.: How to agilely architect an agile architecture. Cutter IT J. **27**, 12–17 (2014)

16. Jeon, S., Han, M., Lee, E., Lee, K.: Quality attribute driven agile development. In: 9th International Conference on Software Engineering Research, Management and Applications (SERA), pp. 203–210. IEEE (2011). https://doi.org/10.1109/SERA.2011.24

17. Nord, R.L., Tomayko, J.E.: Software architecture-centric methods and agile development. IEEE Softw. **23**, 47–53 (2006). https://doi.org/10.1109/MS.2006.54

18. Kanwal, F., Junaid, K., Fahiem, M.A.: A hybrid software architecture evaluation method for FDD-an agile process model. International Conference on Computational Intelligence and Software Engineering (CiSE). IEEE, pp 1–5 (2010). https://doi.org/10.1109/CISE.2010.5676863

19. Santos, N., Pereira, J., Morais, F., Barros, J., Ferreira, N., Machado, R.J.: An agile modeling oriented process for logical architecture design. In: Gulden, J., Reinhartz-Berger, I., Schmidt, R., Guerreiro, S., Guédria, W., Bera, P. (eds.) BPMDS/EMMSAD -2018. LNBIP, vol. 318, pp. 260–275. Springer, Cham (2018). https://doi.org/10.1007/978-3-319-91704-7_17

20. Schwaber, K.: Scrum development process. In: Sutherland, J., Casanave, C., Miller, J., Patel, P., Hollowell, G. (eds.) Business Object Design and Implementation, pp. 117–134. Springer, London (1997). https://doi.org/10.1007/978-1-4471-0947-1_11

21. Mancl, D., Fraser, S., Opdyke, B., et al.: Architecture in an agile world. In: SPLASH/OOPSLA Companion, pp. 289–290. ACM (2009)

22. Coplien, J.O., Bjørnvig, G.: Lean Architecture: For Agile Software Development. Wiley, Hoboken (2011)

23. Zhang, X., Hu, Y., Lu, Y., Gu, J.: University dormitory management system based on agile development architecture. In: IEEE International Conference on Management and Service Science (2011). https://doi.org/10.1109/ICMSS.2011.5998992

24. Harvick, R.: Agile Architecture for Service Oriented Component Driven Enterprises: Encouraging Rapid Application Development using Agile. DataThunder Publishing, Kissimmee (2012)
25. Shariﬂoo, A.A., Saffarian, A.S., Shams, F.: Embedding architectural practices into extreme programming. In: 19th Australian Conference on Software Engineering (ASWEC), pp. 310–319. IEEE (2008). https://doi.org/10.1109/ASWEC.2008.4483219
26. Díaz, J., Pérez, J., Garbajosa, J.: Agile product-line architecting in practice: a case study in smart grids. Inf. Softw. Technol. **56**, 727–748 (2014). https://doi.org/10.1016/j.infsof.2014.01.014
27. Santos, N., Duarte, F.J., Machado, R.J., Fernandes, J.M.: A transformation of business process models into software-executable models using MDA. In: Winkler, D., Biffl, S., Bergsmann, J. (eds.) SWQD 2013. LNBIP, vol. 133, pp. 147–167. Springer, Heidelberg (2013). https://doi.org/10.1007/978-3-642-35702-2_10
28. Neiva, R., Santos, N., Martins, J.C.C., Machado, R.J.: Deriving UML logical architectures of traceability business processes based on a GS1 standard. In: Gervasi, O., et al. (eds.) ICCSA 2015. LNCS, vol. 9158, pp. 528–543. Springer, Cham (2015). https://doi.org/10.1007/978-3-319-21410-8_41
29. Fernandes, J.M., Machado, R.J.: Requirements in Engineering Projects. Springer, Cham (2016). https://doi.org/10.1007/978-3-319-18597-2
30. Douglass, B.: Doing Hard Time: Developing Real-Time Systems with UML, Objects, Frameworks, and Patterns. Addison-Wesley Professional, Boston (1999)
31. Eeles, P., Cripps, P.: The Process of Software Architecting. Pearson Education, London (2009)
32. Kruchten, P.: The 4+1 view model of architecture. IEEE Softw. **12**, 42–50 (1995). https://doi.org/10.1109/52.469759
33. Soni, D., Nord, R.L., Hofmeister, C.: Software architecture in industrial applications. In: 17th International Conference on Software Engineering (ICSE). ACM Press, pp. 196–207 (1995). https://doi.org/10.1145/225014.225033
34. Fong, E.N., Goldfine, A.H.: Information management directions: the integration challenge (1989)
35. Zachman, J.A.: The zachman framework for enterprise architecture (2011)
36. Santos, N., et al.: Specifying software services for fog computing architectures using recursive model transformations. In: Mahmood, Z. (ed.) Fog Computing, pp. 153–181. Springer, Cham (2018). https://doi.org/10.1007/978-3-319-94890-4_8
37. Santos, N., Rodrigues, H., Pereira, J., et al.: UH4SP: a software platform for integrated management of connected smart plants. In: 9th IEEE International Conference on Intelligent Systems (IS). IEEE (2018). https://doi.org/10.1109/IS.2018.8710468
38. Santos, N., Pereira, J., Ferreira, N., Machado, R.J.: Modeling in Agile Software Development: Decomposing Use Cases Towards Logical Architecture Design. In: Kuhrmann, M., et al. (eds.) PROFES 2018. LNCS, vol. 11271, pp. 396–408. Springer, Cham (2018). https://doi.org/10.1007/978-3-030-03673-7_31

Towards Model-Driven Role Engineering in BPM Software Systems

Eduard Babkin[1], Pavel Malyzhenkov[1(✉)],
and Constantine Yavorskiy[2]

[1] Department of Information Systems and Technologies,
National Research University Higher School of Economics,
Bol. Pecherskaya 25, 603155 Nizhny Novgorod, Russia
{eababkin, pmalyzhenkov}@hse.ru
[2] Comindware, Office 5216, 157c5, Dmitrovskoe Highway,
127411 Moscow, Russia
cy@comindware.com

Abstract. This work introduces a new concept of role engineering inside a Model-Driven Engineering modern trend. In case of developing a complex solution comprehensive definition of all needed business roles and their access rights becomes a difficult task. So, the present contribution analyzes different approaches towards the role engineering realized by DEMO and BPMN methodologies based on the Comindware (CBAP) support.

Keywords: Model-driven engineering · DEMO · BPMN · CBAP · Role engineering

1 Introduction

Model-Driven Engineering (MDE) [1–3, 8] is a promising approach to address complexity of software development or configuration of enterprise information systems. Previously proposed third-generation languages demonstrate inability to alleviate this complexity and express domain concepts effectively. The development of MDE technologies combines the following components:

- domain-specific modeling languages (DSML) whose type systems formalize the application structure, behavior, and requirements within particular domains, such as software-defined radios, avionics mission computing, online financial services, warehouse management, or even the domain of middleware platforms. DSMLs are described using metamodels, which define the relationships among concepts in a domain and precisely specify the key semantics and constraints associated with these domain concepts. Developers use DSMLs to build applications using elements of the type system captured by metamodels and express design intent declaratively rather than imperatively;
- transformation engines and generators that analyze certain aspects of models and then synthesize various types of artifacts, such as source code, simulation inputs, XML deployment descriptions, or alternative model representations. The ability to

S. Wrycza and J. Maślankowski (Eds.): SIGSAND/PLAIS 2019, LNBIP 359, pp. 137–146, 2019.
https://doi.org/10.1007/978-3-030-29608-7_11

synthesize artifacts from models helps ensure the consistency between application implementations and analysis information associated with functional and QoS requirements captured by models. This automated transformation process is often referred to as "correct-by-construction," as opposed to conventional handcrafted "construct-by-correction" software development processes that are tedious and error prone. Existing and emerging MDE technologies apply lessons learned from earlier efforts at developing higher-level platform and language abstractions. For example, instead of general-purpose notations that rarely express application domain concepts and design intent, DSMLs can be tailored via metamodeling to precisely match the domain's semantics and syntax. Having graphic elements that relate directly to a familiar domain not only helps flatten learning curves but also helps a broader range of subject matter experts, such as system engineers and experienced software architects, ensure that software systems meet user needs.

To be successful the MDE approach should integrate or adapt bodies of knowledge and techniques available in mature technological spaces. Fortunately, MDE starts to draw the attention of research communities from different fields.

In this work we study opportunities for model-driven engineering in a particular case of configuration of a software platform for business process management (BPM). That kind of software includes a broad range of matured applications [5, 8], which are frequently used now for rapid development of process-oriented information systems in small, medium and even large enterprises. During cooperation with the development team of a leading BPM platform, Comindware Business Application Platform (CBAP) [9], we met a specific manifestation of a generic problem of BPM platforms: lacking modeling support and formal methods for comprehensive and consistent definition of business roles and their access rights within the process definition. That task has significant influence to security, performance and customer experience aspects. Because we pursue a goal to make specification of roles in the context of the BPM platform more predictable and model-based, we offer a special term "Role Engineering" to such kind of activity. In the course of our research we use specific artifacts of CBAP during the initial stage and offer a generic method for mapping between the concepts of the platform-independent enterprise model and configuration parameters needed for role engineering. We use DEMO modeling methodology to design a platform-independent model of the organization and perform the analysis of correspondences between the concepts of DEMO and the concepts of CBAP platform needed during role engineering.

The paper is structured in the following way: Introduction explains the main features of model-driven engineering; Sect. 2 introduces major characteristics of CBAP platform which determine platform-dependent modeling concepts as well as relevant DEMO modeling elements which constitute a basis for platform-independent modeling. Section 3 provides the readers with the concept of role engineering and describes the details of the method proposed for it. Section 5 provides major conclusions and determine future directions of the research.

2 Overview of Platform-Dependent (CBAP) and Platform-Independent (DEMO) Modeling Concepts

Comindware CBAP [9] is one of well-known Business-Process Management (BPM) solutions. This solution allows software engineers to perform low-code design and development of complex domain-oriented applications on the basis of BPMN models and an extensible data model. Comindware CBAP leverages modern and implementation - proven technologies such as HTML, JavaScript and AJAX. The back-end is built using the latest edition of Microsoft.NET Framework. In addition to offering multiple out-of-box configuration capabilities and the Low-code approach, that platform provides deep customization capabilities based on C#. The main elements of CBAP solutions include:

- Process model – represents a connected set of performed activities in BPMN v.2 format.
- Records Templates – define a domain-oriented data model in terms of record types, their attributes and records relationships.
- Forms – define a user-oriented representation of certain record templates for data manipulation during enactment of activities from the process model.
- Roles – specify roles for business-oriented discretion of access rights to the activities, records and forms.

These elements form a platform-dependent meta-model which is instantiated during developing specific domain-oriented artifacts. All elements of particular CBAP solution may be grouped inside the business application.

During our research we consider DEMO [4, 6] modeling artifacts as a platform-independent model. The DEMO concept of actor role is described in detail in [4] where the authority, responsibility and competence for being the executor of a transaction type are defined as an actor role. The competence means the ability of a subject to perform particular production acts as well as the corresponding coordination acts. Moreover, in order to be able to practice one's profession, it is necessary to be appointed or employed by a certain corporate body (a company, a government agency etc.). Through such an act, one gets the authority to practice on behalf of that institution. By virtue of the values and norms of the institution one represents, as well as by virtue of the general cultural values and norms of the society one is member of, one is expected to exert the granted authority in a responsible way. This is what we mean by responsibility. Responsibility becomes manifested primarily in coordination [4].

One of the most important features of DEMO is the distinction between ontological, infological and datalogical transactions. That distinction is known as a organizational theorem [4]: "the organization of an enterprise is a heterogeneous system that is constituted as the layered integration of three homogeneous systems: the B-organization (from Business), the I-organization (from Intellect), and the D-organization (from Document). The relationships among them are that the D-organization supports the

I-organization, and the I-organization supports the B-organization. The integration is established through the cohesive unity of the human being.

Acts like copying, storing, and transmitting data are typical datalogical acts. For example, the act of recording an application for membership in the letter book is considered to be a datalogical act. Next, speaking, listening, writing, and reading are typical datalogical coordination acts. In contrast, an infological production act is an act in which one is not concerned about the form but, instead, about the content of information only. Typical infological acts are inquiring, calculating, and reasoning. As an example, calculating the membership fee is considered to be an infological act. Regarding the coordination between people, formulating thoughts (in written or spoken sentences) and interpreting perceived (through listening or reading) sentences are typical infological coordination acts. An ontological act is an act in which new original things are brought about. Deciding and judging are typical ontological production.

Besides, DEMO shows how much the ontological model of an organization can differ from its implementation. As a general rule, the functionary who performs the promise in a transaction is considered to be the one who is authorized to be executor of that transaction. One becomes authorized for an actor role by being appointed as such. The question is how authority can be transferred by an authorized functionary to someone else and such a transfer of authority is defined as delegation. By this DEMO means that the authorized functionary also remains responsible. So, in the case of authorization, the full responsibility is transferred to the one being authorized; in the case of delegation, the delegator remains ultimately responsible (since he or she is the only authorized one), regardless the agreements that are made between the delegator and the delegate.

3   Role Engineering: Practice and Challenges

For better access control a developer of CBAP-based application should define so-called business roles and their privileges for creation, deletion or modification of certain elements of the CBAP solution. For the purposes of our work we define such design process as **role engineering**.

In a case of developing a complex solution comprehensive definition of all needed business roles and their access rights becomes a difficult task. The challenge consists in the fact that the BPMN standard doesn't define the role concept in some way. Also comprehensive and consistent configuration of role parameters requires deep knowledge of user interfaces and methodological constraints inside the CBAP platform.

For better understanding we use a specific use case of the library service [4]. The corresponding DEMO artifacts for the case described can be designed as follows (Figs. 1, 2, 3).

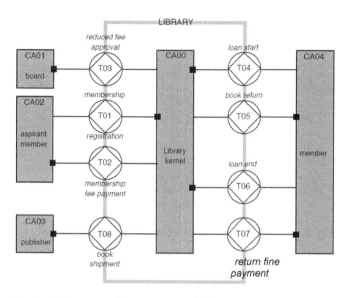

Fig. 1. A Corresponding process model for the case considered [4]

The construction model (CM) of an organization specifies its composition, its environment, and its structure. The composition and the environment are both a set of actor roles. By convention, we will always draw environmental actor roles as composite actor roles, even if we happen to know that an actor role is elementary. The reason for doing this is that generally we do not know whether an environmental actor role is elementary or composite. We start with modeling this kernel as one composite actor role. The resulting CM is usually referred to as the global CM of an organization. Likewise, the CM in which the kernel contains only elementary actor roles is called the detailed CM. The boundary divides the set of all (relevant) actor roles into the composition and the environment.

The numbering of the composite actor roles is arbitrary; it is a convention to number the kernel CA00, such that the environmental actor roles can be numbered CA01, etc. The names of actor roles are not a formal part of a CM; however, using appropriate names may enhance the readability of a diagram considerably. The readability is also enhanced by mentioning the transaction names next to the transaction symbols. The actor role CA02 (aspirant member) represents the persons who want to become member of the library. Obviously, it is the initiator of T01 (membership registration). CA02 is also considered to be the executor of T02 (membership fee payment). The actor role CA04 (member) represents the actual members of the library. It is the initiator of T04 (loan start) and the executor of T05 (book return).

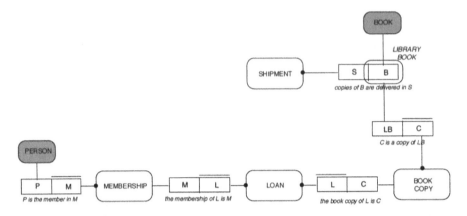

Fig. 2. A Corresponding OFD model for the case considered [4]

property type	object class	scale
date_of_birth	PERSON	JULIAN DATE
age (*)	PERSON	NUMBER
#days_overdue (*)	LOAN	NUMBER
incurred_fine (*)	LOAN	EURO
minimal_age	YEAR	NUMBER
standard_fee	YEAR	EURO
reduced_fee	YEAR	EURO
normal_loan_period	YEAR	NUMBER
max_copies_in_loan	YEAR	NUMBER
daily_late_fine	YEAR	EURO
#books_of_shipment	SHIPMENT	NUMBER
#books_in_loan (*)	MEMBERSHIP	NUMBER

Fig. 3. A Corresponding OPL model for the case considered [4]

If we aim at developing a corresponding business application for CBAP the following artifacts should be developed (Table 1):

Table 1. Platform-dependent artifacts for CBAP Application

Meta-model element	Instances
Records	Book, Shipment, Book Copy, Loan, Membership, Person[a]
Forms	Fill Membership Registration, Fill Reduced Fee Application, Book Shipment Form, Loan Start, Loan End, Fill Return Fine Form
Processes	Reduced Fee Approval, Membership Registration, Membership Payment, Book Shipment, Loan Start, Book Return, Loan End, Return Fine Payment

[a]A person CBAP record is a virtual one – needed data about persons are available from the system catalog.

We also need to perform role engineering to separate different groups of users and assign them only the access rights which are really needed for accomplishment of the process tasks.

According to the DEMO model the following actors are distinguished: aspirant member, board, member, library kernel.

In our approach we propose to apply a direct mapping between DEMO actors and business roles of CBAP-platform. That design choice corresponds to the authorization of a specified actor to fulfill the transaction. Delegation of transaction fulfillment to the infological level of transactions can also be considered. However practical implementation of such method in CBAP requires modification of functionality.

According to our approach a designer of CBAP application should specify business-roles according to the authorization of DEMO actors. CBAP provides a designer with a special web-interface for assigning certain privileges to the corresponding business-roles (Fig. 4):

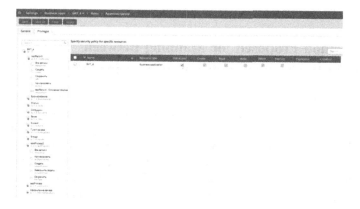

Fig. 4. A Web-based interface for role creation and specification

In addition the same business roles can be used for specification of BPMN swimlines during specification of BPMN diagrams. Figure 5 shows a corresponding BPMN diagram for several DEMO transactions.

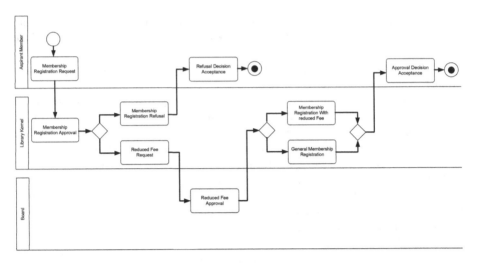

Fig. 5. A Corresponding BPMN process model in CBAP for DEMO transactions

4 The Method Proposed for Mapping Between Platform-Independent and Platform Dependent Models

In our method of role engineering we follow generic principles of model-driven design and aim at automatic engineering of business roles and their access rights for CBAP solutions. We use DEMO modeling methodology to design a platform-independent model of the organization and perform the analysis of correspondences between the concepts of DEMO and the concepts of CBAP platform needed during role engineering.

The ontological model of library is really and fully abstracted from the current way in which it operates. It does not contain organizational functions, like secretary and administrator and members, or references to persons. It also does not contain any infological or datalogical things: no computing, no inquiring, no letter book, no register, etc. Moreover, it completely abstracts from the way in which the fulfillers of the distinguished actor roles communicate: no letters, no telephone calls, etc. These properties, of course, make the ontological model very stable. A new organizational structure will not change the ontology; nor will replacing letters by e-mails; nor will replacing the register book by a database, and so on.

Joint analysis of DEMO models and the elements of the CBAP web-interface leads to the conclusion, that the following correspondence rules between DEMO models and CBAP elements are valid in general (Table 2).

Table 2. Meta-modeling mapping rules proposed

Artifact of the DEMO meta-model	CBAP artifact
Actor	Business-role
Initiator of transaction	Permission to create a process-related record
Executor of transaction	Permission to read/write create a process-related record
Element of OFD/OFL	Specific record template
Process model, construction model	Specific process model

If we apply the rules above to our case study the following results of role engineering can be produced (Tables 3, 4).

Table 3. The results of the mapping application

CBAP meta-model artifacts	CBAP model artifacts
Business-role	Library Kernel, Aspirant Member, Member, Board, Publisher
Record template	Book, Shipment, Book Copy, Loan, Membership

Table 4. The results of the role engineering

Roles/Records	Book	Shipment	Book Copy	Loan	Membership
Library Kernel	CRUD	RU	CRUD	RU	RU
Aspirant Member	R				CR
Member	R			CU	
Board					RU
Publisher		C			

Permission Legend: C – create; R – read; U – update; D – delete.

The results of mapping application, corresponding BPMN diagrams and role engineering artifacts were created in CBAP using a designer web-interface. During practical validation of the CBAP business application with such access rights it was affirmed, that all users have needed access rights. At the same time, their rights prevent unauthorized access to CBAP elements outside the framework of the process.

5 Discussion and Conclusions

That result shows applicability of mapping between DEMO models and CBAP BPM platform elements during role engineering. Proposed mapping rules provide a complete and consistent mechanism for model-driven role engineering, and open practical opportunities for automation of that process. Moreover, the table with the rights description provides considerable assistance to the architects of the CBAP solution. They can use only this scheme and not thoroughly study the business process. Besides the table itself can be constructed automatically.

Proposed approach may be extended to more sophisticated cases of authorization-delegation chains, when, in terms of DEMO modeling, the ontological level of organization is further supported by infological and datalogical levels. Such nesting of different organizational levels is known as realization [4]. In order to support multi-layer realization a considerable number of CBAP solution functions should be modified.

Our next stage of the research will be focused on implementation of the mapping rules programmatically inside a problem-specific modeling environment. Besides, another research direction could be represented by the application of this methodology to the assessment of process modeling tools [7].

References

1. Brambilla, M., Cabot, J., Wimmer, M.: Model-Driven Software Engineering in Practice. Morgan & Claypool Publishers, San Rafael (2017)
2. Brouwers, N., Hamilton, M., Kurtev, I., You, L.: Language architecture: an architecture language for model-driven engineering. In: MODELSWARD 2017. Science and Technology Publications, Lda (2017)
3. De Lara, J., Guerra, E., Cuadrado, J.S.: Model-driven engineering with domain-specific meta-modelling languages. Softw. Syst. Model. **14**, 429–459 (2015)
4. Dietz, J.L.G.: Enterprise Ontology: Theory and Methodology. Springer, Heidelberg (2006). https://doi.org/10.1007/3-540-33149-2
5. Lohmann, P., Zur Muehlen, M.: Business process management skills and roles: an investigation of the demand and supply side of BPM professionals. In: Motahari-Nezhad, H.R., Recker, J., Weidlich, M. (eds.) BPM 2015. LNCS, vol. 9253, pp. 317–332. Springer, Cham (2015). https://doi.org/10.1007/978-3-319-23063-4_22
6. Mráz, O., Náplava, P., Pergl, R., Skotnica, M.: Converting DEMO PSI transaction pattern into BPMN: a complete method. In: Aveiro, D., Pergl, R., Guizzardi, G., Almeida, J.P., Magalhães, R., Lekkerkerk, H. (eds.) EEWC 2017. LNBIP, vol. 284, pp. 85–98. Springer, Cham (2017). https://doi.org/10.1007/978-3-319-57955-9_7
7. Pavlicek, J., Pavlickova, P.: Methods for evaluating the quality of process modelling tools. In: Pergl, R., Babkin, E., Lock, R., Malyzhenkov, P., Merunka, V. (eds.) EOMAS 2018. LNBIP, vol. 332, pp. 171–177. Springer, Cham (2018). https://doi.org/10.1007/978-3-030-00787-4_12
8. Uhl, A., Gollenia, L.A.: A Handbook of Business Transformation Management Methodology. Routledge, London (2016)
9. E-resources. https://www.comindware.com/

Communication and Documentation Practices in Agile Requirements Engineering: A Survey in Polish Software Industry

Aleksander Jarzębowicz$^{(\boxtimes)}$ ⓘ and Natalia Sitko

Department of Software Engineering, Faculty of Electronics,
Telecommunications and Informatics, Gdańsk University of Technology,
Gdańsk, Poland
olek@eti.pg.edu.pl

Abstract. Requirements engineering, system analysis and other analytical activities form the basis of every IT project. Such activities are not clearly defined in Agile development methods, but it does not mean that they are absent in an agile project. The aim of our work was to determine which practices related to requirements-related communication and which requirements documenting techniques are used in agile software projects. For this reason we carried out a survey study targeting agile practitioners from Polish IT industry. The paper presents survey results, discusses the noticed differences with respect to the general Agile values and principles and provides a comparison to results of similar studies described in the related work. The main observation about communication practices is that frequent, face to face communication is the most common, but many respondents also declare use of other, remote communication means or exchanging SRS documents. The investigation of requirements documentation techniques revealed differences between the techniques used while describing requirements for developers and those used to elicit requirements from stakeholders and to comprehend them.

Keywords: Requirements engineering · Software projects · Agile requirements · Agile development · Scrum

1 Introduction

To provide an effective solution, it is first necessary to understand the problem, thus analytical activities form the basis of every IT project. Such activities are known under the names of requirements engineering (RE), business analysis (BA) or system analysis (SA), which somewhat differ with respect to scope and focus, but all include capturing and exploring the needs of the customer and relevant stakeholders. A large body of knowledge is available in e.g. international standards [1] and industrial guides [2–4]. Such sources provide comprehensive guidelines on processes, roles, techniques and recommended practices. It is worth to note an increased interest of the industry, especially on the topics of RE and BA, which resulted in publishing the abovementioned guides in recent years.

© Springer Nature Switzerland AG 2019
S. Wrycza and J. Maślankowski (Eds.): SIGSAND/PLAIS 2019, LNBIP 359, pp. 147–158, 2019.
https://doi.org/10.1007/978-3-030-29608-7_12

At the same time, in the last 10–15 years the IT industry has increasingly adopted Agile development approach [5], which is currently commonly used in software projects worldwide [6]. The generic Agile approach and particular Agile development methods like Scrum or Extreme Programming do not distinguish RE, BA, SA or other analytical activities as a separate phase, area or discipline of a software project. Moreover, the Agile values suggest "light" processes and minimizing software project artefacts (documentation). As analysis is not emphasized, an initial impression can arise that RE is not important in agile projects, especially considering that e.g. Scrum or XP do not define any "analyst" role and encourage the direct, face to face communication between customer representatives and all members of the development team. It would be a wrong conclusion though, as Agile and RE practices can and should be used together [7–9]. Moreover, in practice the role of an analyst is often present in agile software projects and is of crucial importance [10, 11].

The term of "Agile Requirements Engineering" (ARE) was defined [12] to describe RE activities and practices tailored to be used in an Agile context. ARE expands the guidelines included in Agile methods like Scrum, by covering in more detail RE practices (which are not comprehensively defined in those methods). In some cases where such guidelines turn out to be insufficient in practice, ARE provides additional solutions. For example, an assumption that a single customer representative (covering all stakeholders' viewpoints) would be available to work on site with development team on daily basis is often hard to satisfy [12]. A possible solution is that an analyst serves as an "interface" between stakeholders from the customer side and the development team from the supplier side. Another example is the problem of minimal documentation and simplified representation of requirements like user stories [13], which can e.g. drive an analyst to create user stories for the inclusion in Product Backlog, but additionally document requirements using another specification technique that allows him/her a better comprehension of requirements and facilitates cooperation with stakeholders. On the other hand, ARE introduces concepts differing from more traditional RE e.g. agile requirements quality criteria [14] or less formal RE techniques including collaborative games [15].

To summarize - ARE uses its dedicated practices [13], utilizes so called agile mindset [16] and encounters some specific problems and challenges, different from RE in projects that use plan-driven development methods [17]. An ongoing research efforts are dedicated to both ARE practices [18–21] and challenges [18, 20, 22].

In our research we intended to identify the status quo of RE practices in agile software projects conducted in an IT industry in Poland. A number of surveys on Agile adoption in the industry (addressing the topic of RE or at least including it within scope) were conducted in several countries [6, 20, 23, 24]. However, to the best of our knowledge, there are no scientific papers about such study in the context of Polish IT industry. It is a research gap we intended to address. In particular, the work we report here focused on the following research questions:

- RQ1 – Which practices related to cooperation and communication between various project participants are used in agile software projects in Polish IT industry?
- RQ2 – Which requirements documentation techniques are used in agile software projects in Polish IT industry?
- RQ3 – Are such practices and techniques consistent with Agile guidelines?

This paper is structured as follows. Section 2 outlines the way we designed and conducted the industrial survey study. In Sect. 3 the results of this study are presented, together with the accompanying discussion, moreover threats to validity are addressed. In Sect. 4 we summarize related work and compare our results to those presented in the literature. The paper is concluded in Sect. 5.

2   Survey Study

We planned and designed a questionnaire-based survey study investigating the RE practices in agile software development projects. We defined our target population as the participants of agile projects conducted in Polish IT industry. We did not limit our focus to any specific domains nor types of software products. We used a web questionnaire developed using GoogleForms[1]. The language used was Polish, in this paper we provide English translations of questions and answers. The questionnaire consisted of two main parts: questions about respondent's background and demographics (e.g. role/responsibility, experience in industrial agile projects, Agile methods used) and questions about RE practices and techniques the respondent uses in projects he/she participates. The following questions about communication and requirements documentation were included:

- (Q1) What is the source of requirements in most agile projects?
- (Q2) How frequent is the contact between analysts (or other development team members) and customer representatives?
- (Q3) How do analysts cooperate with customer representatives?
- (Q4) How are the requirements communicated to the development team?
- (Q5) Which techniques do analysts use to document requirements for the purposes of comprehending them and analyst-customer cooperation?
- (Q6) Which techniques do analysts use to document requirements for the purpose of analyst-development team cooperation?

All of questions Q1–Q6 were a multiple choice questions. The available responses included pre-defined answers prepared on the basis of literature review (to cover all popular practices) and additionally "Other" answer, followed by a text field to input additional feedback. The questionnaire was developed iteratively and reviewed several times, finally a pilot study involving 3 people belonging to the target population was conducted as the final verification activity.

We are not aware of any means we could recruit a representative sample of the investigated target population in a systematic way. As result, we could only rely on non-systematic sampling methods, and therefore we used convenience sampling. We distributed invitations to participate in our survey to Agile interest groups in social network media (LinkedIn, Facebook, GoldenLine). We also sent direct messages with invitations using the contacts established at the software engineering beIT[2] conference

---

[1] https://www.google.com/forms/about/.

[2] www.konferencjabeit.pl/.

and practitioners identified by their CV contents at LinkedIn. The survey was anonymous, no questions about respondent's identity were asked.

The responses were gathered in the period of April–June 2018. We verified them against pre-defined criteria and removed 4 of them that were either incomplete (only some questions answered) or indicated that the respondent had no industrial experience (e.g. participated in agile projects done as part of university studies only). After verification, the number of responses left was 69.

The responses were then processed and analyzed. Visualizations depicting the distribution of answers are included in Sect. 3. We also paid attention to potential differences in answers regarding less experienced respondents (up to 2 years of experience in agile development) and analysts (and Product Owners), who are more committed to RE and can be considered more aware of RE practices. We do not provide any separate visualization of answers provided by such sub-groups, but in cases such differences were spotted, we mention them while discussing results.

After the survey was completed and its results processed, we invited two experienced analysts (of 10 and 15 years of experience in RE and BA, respectively) to review the results with us and share their interpretations, especially in cases the results were found surprising. Their feedback is also included in Sect. 3 discussion.

3   Results

As already mentioned, after removing questionable answers, we were left with the data provided by 69 respondents. The background questions allowed us to determine some context information about the sample of population we received responses from. Most of our respondents worked as developers (49,3%), followed by analysts (36,2%). The remaining 14,5% identified themselves mostly as Product Owners and project managers. It is not surprising that majority of respondents were developers as it is the most common role in agile projects (and not only agile), however the percentage of analysts seems to be higher than in most teams and companies – this can be explained though by the fact that they were probably the most interested in the survey on ARE.

The experience in agile development the respondents declared is shown on the left part of Fig. 1. About half of them had a limited experience (less than 2 years) thus their answers can be challenged as less reliable, however we decided to use them, but with additional attention to spot anomalies (questions for which answers of less experienced respondents were significantly different than the answers of remaining survey participants). About 40% declared experience between 2 and 5 years and only a small group claimed more than 5 years in agile development. This can be explained in two ways: first - that Agile adoption as the "mainstream" approach in Polish industry can be dated only a few years back; second – that more experienced people have more professional responsibilities and less time to spare for answering survey questionnaires. As for Agile development methods, depicted on the right side of Fig. 1, it is clear that the most popular method is Scrum. Another popular method is Kanban, which however is used together with Scrum, not as the only development method followed.

In the following part of this section we report answers to questions about agile requirements processes and techniques (Q1–Q6). Please note, that they were multiple

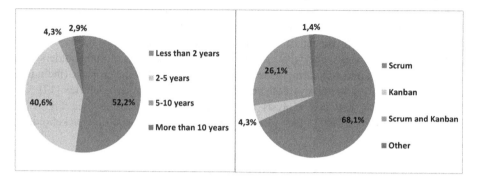

Fig. 1. Survey respondents' experience in agile development (left) and Agile methods used by them (right).

choice questions, therefore we use numbers not percentages when presenting them.

According to our respondents, the most common source of requirements in agile projects are stakeholders - people from whom the requirements are elicited. It is

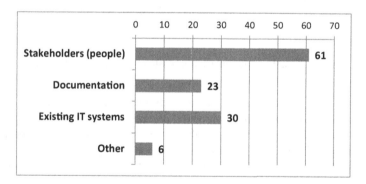

Fig. 2. Sources of requirements in agile projects (Q1).

interesting though that almost half of respondents identified existing IT systems as requirement sources and one third the written documentation (see Fig. 2). This deviates to some extent from Agile values which emphasize direct, face to face communication, but can likely be attributed to the reality software developers meet – legacy systems without any person able to explain how they were designed, "terms of reference" documents required by law in projects in public sector etc.

As shown in Fig. 3, most of respondents (almost half) declare that the contact with customer representatives is maintained on daily basis, which is consistent with Agile approach and its close collaboration themes. Nevertheless, the remaining respondents admitted that such contact is less frequent e.g. before and/or after each sprint/iteration.

We also received a number of "Other" choices, followed by free text answers, most of which declared that such contact takes place: when needed, once a week, a few times a week or depending on the project/the customer. The possible explanation is that when analyst acts as a Scrum's Product Owner (or supports the Product Owner) he/she is responsible for explaining requirements to developers as well as answering their questions and the involvement of customer representatives or other business stake-holders is not necessary every day. Moreover, low availability of stakeholders is a commonly encountered requirements-related problem in software projects (including agile ones), according to surveys both in Poland [25] and in other countries [17].

The cooperation between analysts and customer representatives (see Fig. 4) is mostly based on direct, face to face meetings with individual or multiple stakeholders,

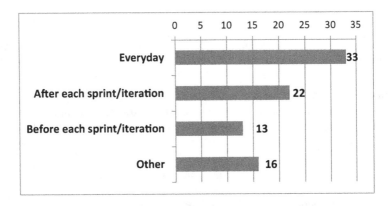

Fig. 3. Frequency of contact with customer representatives (Q2).

which fits well into Agile "people and interactions" value. Still, e-mails, teleconfer-ences and phone calls are quite commonly practiced, which can stem from stake-holders' low availability or from the fact that to answer a well-defined question it is not necessary to arrange a meeting. Interestingly, over one third of our respondents work in agile projects using software requirements specification (SRS) documents, shared with customer representatives.

An essential task in analyst-developer cooperation is the communication of requirements to the developers, in order to be implemented. The answers we collected (Fig. 5) are in line with Scrum recommended practices – the requirements are com-municated directly at the meetings and registered in Product Backlog, moreover ded-icated supporting tools like Confluence[3] are used. A group of respondents (of about the same size as in the previous question) declares using SRS documents though.

As for requirement documentation techniques used in agile projects, we asked two separate questions (Q5 and Q6). The rationale was that we intended to verify whether different documentation techniques are used for different purposes. Agile methods like

---

[3] https://www.atlassian.com/software/confluence.

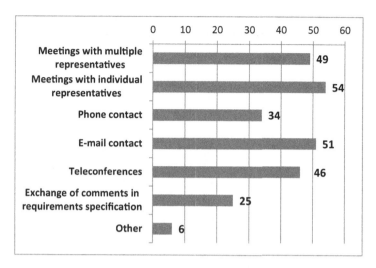

Fig. 4. The means of cooperation between analysts and customer representatives (Q3).

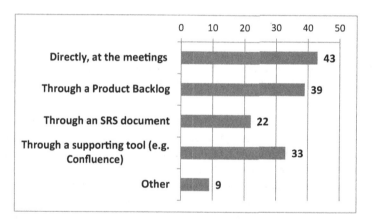

Fig. 5. The means of communicating requirements to the development team (Q4).

Scrum make use of simplified representations of requirements (user stories, features) and it is likely that such representations would be delivered to developers, included in Product Backlog and, when necessary, such requirements would be refined and explained as part of a meeting and direct communication. We were however curious if other documentation techniques are used by analysts for the purpose of comprehending requirements (a necessary condition to be able to explain them to developers) and/or for the purpose of the cooperation between the analyst and customer representatives (e.g. requirements elicitation or validation).

As in both questions the respondents could choose from the same set of techniques, we present answers to Q5 and Q6 jointly in Fig. 6. The results seem to confirm our hypothesis – user stories are more often created for developers than as a working

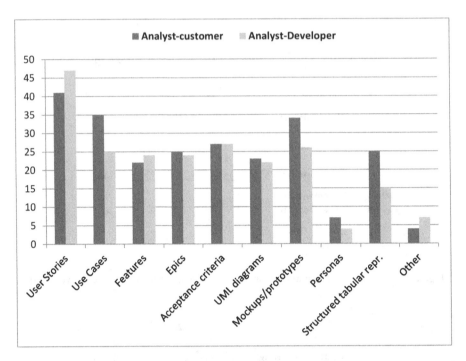

Fig. 6. The comparison of requirements documentation techniques used by analysts in cooperation with customer representatives and with development team (Q5 and Q6).

representation of requirements used by analysts when cooperating with customer representatives. For the latter purpose, analysts tend to choose use cases, mockups/prototypes and structured tabular representations of requirements. It is also worth mentioning, that in responses given by analysts and Product Owners only, the most common documentation technique used in analyst-customer cooperation were mockups/prototypes, followed by use cases and user stories.

We are aware of several limitations of our study and potential threats to validity, they are discussed below with respect to 3 main categories of threats.

Construct Validity: Agile practices can differ among organizations, moreover the names used to describe them can differ as well. The possible threats are that we could omit some relevant practices/techniques (and not include them among predefined answers) and that the names we used could not be clear to our respondents. We mitigated the first threat by preparing the questionnaire on the basis of a literature review and by providing the opportunity to enter manually another answer ("Other" option). We have not noticed any pattern in manually entered answers that the same themes were repeated by numerous respondents. The second threat of possible misunderstanding of terms used was mitigated by several reviews and corrections of the questionnaire, the reviews were conducted not only by us, but also by pilot respondents.

Internal Validity: The main threat we recognize here is the participation of people were not qualified enough to provide information we expected – it was mitigated by reviewing answers and removing those indicating lack of industrial experience. The answers were also checked for signs of fatigue or lack of commitment, but we did not found any.

External Validity: The convenience sampling we used to involve survey respondents and the particular actions we took for this purpose (using social media groups, direct messages, respondents' anonymity) do not allow us to determine exactly how many people read our invitations and what subgroup of them participated in the survey. It is possible that a bias concerning respondents' representativeness was introduced here i.e. that people of a given profile were more likely to participate than others. A significant share of analysts and Product Owners as well as practitioners with low experience seem to confirm possibility of this threat. It is the threat we have to accept and acknowledge.

4 Related Work

Although a significant body of knowledge on ARE exists, we will only refer to directly related work. A more comprehensive review of ARE research can be found in systematic mapping studies by Heikkilä et al. [12], Inayat et al. [18] or Schön et al. [19].

Cao and Ramesh [13] described 7 ARE practices most common to 16 software organizations they analyzed, together with discussion of benefits and challenges of each practice. Among those practices were: face-to-face communication, iterative RE and prototyping, which correspond to our findings. It is also worth to note that heavy or medium usage of prototyping was reported by 11 organizations, while the remaining ones did not use it at all, which resembles our results on mackups/prototypes.

Kassab [6] presented the results of a U.S. survey on RE practices. It was not limited to agile software development, but some results concern agile practices/techniques. Kassab notes the emergence of user stories and informal requirements representations and at the same time a slight decline of prototyping (even in agile projects). Simply comparing the numbers (response ratios), his and our results look similar, however, as he did not distinguish the purpose of the documentation techniques, we cannot make a more detailed comparison of our findings on RQ2 and his work.

Jarzębowicz and Połocka [26] focused on requirements documentation techniques and their applicability to different software project contexts. The respondents of the survey they conducted, selected: user stories, use cases (and scenarios), prototypes and process models as the techniques most applicable to projects developed using Agile methods. All techniques, except the last one, appeared in the questionnaire described in this paper and were among the most commonly used techniques, which suggest that these two studies corroborate each other.

Wagner et al. [20] report partial results of a large family of surveys dedicated to RE practices and problems, focusing on the data provided by respondents working in agile setting. They enumerate interviews, prototyping and facilitated meetings (including workshops) as most popular techniques of cooperating with customer representatives to elicit requirements. As for requirements documentation techniques, they report: free-form textual domain/business process models, free-form textual structured requirements lists and use case models as most popular techniques, while formal and semi-formal models are rarely used.

Ochodek and Kopczyńska [21] conducted an international survey on ARE practices with a significantly wider scope of processes and practices than our study. They processed the results to create the ranking of relative importance of the practices. Among practices corresponding to our study's scope, "Available/on-site customer" and "Provide easy access to requirements" were ranked as most important, while "Notation easy to understand by all stakeholders" and "Write short, negotiable requirements" were considered as significantly less essential, which seems to be in line with our findings.

5 Conclusions

In this paper we reported the research study aimed at investigating requirements-related communication practices and requirement documentation techniques used in agile software development projects in Polish IT industry.

As for RQ1 and communication practices, we can observe that frequent, face to face communication is the most common, however many respondents also declare use of remote communication means or exchanging SRS documents. Investigation of RQ2 and requirements documentation techniques revealed differences between the techniques used while describing requirements for developers (user stories) and those used to elicit requirements from stakeholders and to comprehend them (mockups/prototypes, use cases and structured tabular descriptions). To answer RQ3, we identified some discrepancies between the theory (Agile values and principles) and reality (survey answers). We believe our research can have some implications.

The implications for practitioners – the practitioners can evaluate their current agile requirements engineering practices/techniques and position themselves with respect to the picture of Polish IT industry that was revealed by survey results. This can also be an input to decisions about introducing other practices/techniques to their agile development processes.

The implications for researchers – despite the fact that many surveys and other research studies investigating the practice of agile requirements engineering were conducted, none of them was dedicated to Polish IT industry. This can aid researchers, especially related to the domestic IT industry to steer their research and investigate further e.g. the benefits, limitations and challenges of particular practices and techniques. These are also the possible directions of further research we are considering ourselves.

References

1. ISO/IEC/IEEE: ISO/IEC/IEEE 29148:2011. Systems and software engineering life cycle processes. Requirements engineering (2011)

2. International Institute of Business Analysis: Business Analysis Body of Knowledge (BABOK Guide) version 3 (2015)
3. Project Management Institute: Business Analysis for Practitioners A Practice Guide (2015)
4. International Requirements Engineering Board: IREB CPRE Foundation Level Syllabus ver. 2.2.2 (2017)
5. Fowler, M., Highsmith, J.: The agile manifesto. Softw. Dev. **9**(8), 28–35 (2001)
6. Kassab, M.: The changing landscape of requirements engineering practices over the past decade. In 5th International Workshop on Empirical Requirements Engineering (EmpiRE), pp. 1–8. IEEE (2015)
7. Paetsch, F., Eberlein, A., Maurer, F.: Requirements engineering and agile software development. In: 12th IEEE International Workshops on Enabling Technologies: Infrastructure for Collaborative Enterprises (WETICE), pp. 308–313. IEEE (2003)
8. Sillitti, A., Ceschi, M., Russo, B., Succi, G.: Managing uncertainty in requirements: a survey in documentation-driven and agile companies. In: 11th IEEE International Software Metrics Symposium (METRICS 2005), pp. 10–17. IEEE (2005)
9. International Institute of Business Analysis: Agile Extension to the BABOK Guide, Version 2 (2017)
10. Gregorio, D.: How the business analyst supports and encourages collaboration on agile projects. In: IEEE International Systems Conference (SysCon), pp. 1–4. IEEE (2012)
11. Rogers, G.: RE in Agile Projects: Survey Results, Requirements Engineering Magazine. IREB (2016). https://re-magazine.ireb.org/articles/re-in-agile-projects-survey-results
12. Heikkilä, V.T., Damian, D., Lassenius, C., Paasivaara, M.: A mapping study on requirements engineering in agile software development. In: 41st Euromicro Conference on Software Engineering and Advanced Applications, pp. 199–207. IEEE (2015)
13. Cao, L., Ramesh, B.: Agile requirements engineering practices: An empirical study. IEEE Softw. **25**(1), 60–67 (2008)
14. Heck, P., Zaidman, A.: A systematic literature review on quality criteria for agile requirements specifications. Softw. Qual. J. **26**(1), 127–160 (2018)
15. Przybyłek, A., Zakrzewski, M.: Adopting collaborative games into agile requirements engineering. In: 13th International Conference on Evaluation of Novel Approaches to Software Engineering (ENASE 2018), pp. 54–64 (2018)
16. Miler, J., Gaida, P.: On the agile mindset of an effective team – an industrial opinion survey. In: Federated Conference on Computer Science and Information Systems (FedCSIS 2019), Leipzig, Germany (2019)
17. Méndez Fernández, D., et al.: Naming the pain in requirements engineering: contemporary problems, causes, and effects in practice. Empir. Softw. Eng. **22**, 2298–2338 (2017). https://doi.org/10.1007/s10664-016-9451-7
18. Inayat, I., Salim, S.S., Marczak, S., Daneva, M., Shamshirband, S.: A systematic literature review on agile requirements engineering practices and challenges. Comput. Hum. Behav. **51**, 915–929 (2015)
19. Schön, E.M., Thomaschewski, J., Escalona, M.J.: Agile requirements engineering: a systematic literature review. Comput. Stand. Interfaces **49**, 79–91 (2017)
20. Wagner, S., Méndez Fernández, D., Kalinowski, M., Felderer, M.: Agile requirements engineering in practice: status quo and critical problems. CLEI Electron. J. **21**(1), 15 (2018)
21. Ochodek, M., Kopczyńska, S.: Perceived importance of agile requirements engineering practices – a survey. J. Syst. Softw. **143**, 29–43 (2018)
22. Alsaqaf, W., Daneva, M., Wieringa, R.: Quality requirements challenges in the context of large-scale distributed agile: an empirical study. In: Proceedings of 24th Requirements Engineering: Foundation for Software Quality Conference (REFSQ), pp. 139–154 (2018)

23. Rodríguez, P., Markkula, J., Oivo, M., Turula, K.: Survey on agile and lean usage in Finnish software industry. In: ACM-IEEE International Symposium on Empirical Software Engineering and Measurement (ESEM), pp. 139–148. IEEE (2012)

24. Diel, E., Bergmann, M., Marczak, S., Luciano, E.: What is agile, which practices are used, and which skills are necessary according to Brazilian professionals: findings of an initial survey. In: 6th Brazilian Workshop on Agile Methods (WBMA), pp. 18–24. IEEE (2015)

25. Jarzębowicz, A., Ślesiński, W.: What is troubling IT analysts? a survey report from Poland on requirements-related problems. In: Kosiuczenko, P., Zieliński, Z. (eds.) KKIO 2018. AISC, vol. 830, pp. 3–19. Springer, Cham (2019). https://doi.org/10.1007/978-3-319-99617-2_1

26. Jarzębowicz, A., Połocka, K.: Selecting requirements documentation techniques for software projects: a survey study. In: Federated Conference on Computer Science and Information Systems (FedCSIS 2017), pp. 1205–1214 (2017)

Author Index

Babkin, Eduard   137

Dori, Dov   37

Elnagar, Samaa   3

Faustino, João   77
Ferreira, Nuno   121

Jarzębowicz, Aleksander   147
Jbara, Ahmad   37

Kelsey, Karishma   62
Kirikova, Marite   48
Kohen, Hanan   37
Kolkowska, Ella   48
Kritzinger, Elmarie   91
Kuciapski, Michał   20

Lech, Przemysław   12
Levi-Soskin, Natali   37

Machado, Ricardo J.   121
Malyzhenkov, Pavel   137

Pereira, Rúben   77
Prates, Luís   77

Sandhu, Ramandeep Kaur   105
Santos, Nuno   121
Scholtz, Dorothy   91
Shaoul, Ron   37
Silva, Miguel   77
Sitko, Natalia   147
Soja, Ewa   48
Soja, Piotr   48
Stanley-Brown, Josephine   105

Weichbroth, Paweł   20
Weistroffer, Heinz Roland   3, 105

Yavorskiy, Constantine   137

Zaliwski, Andrew   62

Printed in the United States
By Bookmasters